Praise for *Feeding You Lies*

"There are 3,000 food additives in our food supply, many of which have not been tested for safety, and the average American consumes three to five pounds of these chemicals a year. In *Feeding You Lies*, Vani Hari pulls back the veil of , deception by the food industry, scientists, and the media designed to manipulate us and ignore the unnecessary harms in our food supply. The deep investigation of the actions of the media, food companies, and science to suppress the truth will shock you, make you stop and consider what you put in your mouth, as well as empower you with the tools and strategies to protect yourself from bad foods and lies. If you eat, read this book."

— **Mark Hyman, M.D.**, #1 *New York Times* best-selling author of *Food: What the Heck Should I Eat?* and director, Cleveland Clinic Center for Functional Medicine

"A tangled web of deception is unraveled in this provocative page-turner! My eyes are now wide open thanks to Vani's tireless investigative work to expose the truth about the food we eat."

— **Lewis Howes**, *New York Times* best-selling author of *The School of Greatness*

"With all the wrongdoings exposed in this book, it's no wonder that so many are confused about what to eat! You'll never walk into a grocery store with the same outlook after learning the revealing information presented in this thoughtful read."

— **Frank Lipman, M.D.**, *New York Times* best-selling author of *The New Health Rules* and *How to Be Well*

"Our food is making many of us fat, sick, and miserable; but it's making certain companies billions of dollars. To us, the fact that disease rates are skyrocketing is a matter of life or death; but to them, it's just a PR problem. This magnificent book by the courageous and brilliant food activist Vani Hari shows you how to see through the lies, how to know the truth about what you are eating, and how to feed yourself and your family foods that will truly nourish your body, your mind, and your spirit."

— **John Robbins**, co-founder and president of Food Revolution Network and best-selling author of *Diet for a New America*

"The tobacco industry survived for decades by marketing 'doubt as our product.' Big Food is following in their footsteps. I am grateful to Vani Hari for exposing the abuse of trust and the descending health of the public at the hands of Big Food. · Her simple Three Question Detox is a platform to upgrade the health of your family. Everyone should read this book."

— **Joel Kahn, M.D., FACC**, clinical professor of medicine, Wayne State University School of Medicine, and author of *The Plant-Based Solution*

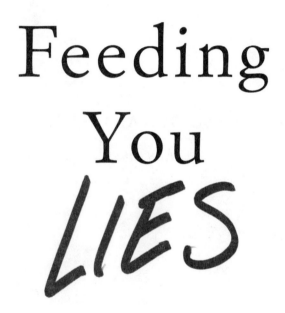

Feeding You LIES

ALSO BY VANI HARI

The Food Babe Way

■ ■ ■

Feeding You *LIES*

HOW TO UNRAVEL THE FOOD INDUSTRY'S PLAYBOOK AND RECLAIM YOUR HEALTH

Vani Hari

HAY HOUSE, INC.
Carlsbad, California • New York City
London • Sydney • New Delhi

Published in the United States by: Hay House, Inc.: www.hayhouse.com®
Published in Australia by: Hay House Australia Pty. Ltd.: www.hayhouse.com.au
Published in the United Kingdom by: Hay House UK, Ltd.: www.hayhouse.co.uk
Published in India by: Hay House Publishers India: www.hayhouse.co.in

Cover design: Samantha Russo • *Interior design:* Nick C. Welch
Indexer: Jay Kreider

Library of Congress Cataloging-in-Publication Data

Names: Hari, Vani, author.
Title: Feeding you lies : how to unravel the food industry's playbook and
  reclaim your health / Vani Hari.
Description: 1st edition. | Carlsbad, California : Hay House, Inc., 2019 |
  Includes bibliographical references and index.
Identifiers: LCCN 2018049666| ISBN 9781401954543 (hardcover : alk. paper) |
  ISBN 9781401954550 (ebook)
Subjects: LCSH: Nutrition. | Food.
Classification: LCC RA784 .H364 2019 | DDC 613.2--dc23 LC record available at
  https://lccn.loc.gov/2018049666

Hardcover ISBN: 978-1-4019-5454-3
e-book ISBN: 978-1-4019-5455-0

10 9 8 7 6 5 4 3 2
1st edition, February 2019

Printed in the United States of America

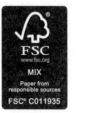
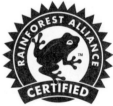

To my daughter,
Harley,
and my husband,
Finley

■ ■ ■

Contents

Introduction

I was sitting on a plane, heading to New York City for one of the most important interviews of my life. *The New York Times* had asked to do a profile piece on me, highlighting the work I'd been doing in regard to dangerous food additives and dishonest tactics used by the Big Food industry.

The previous 12 months had been a whirlwind. Subway restaurants agreed to remove the "yoga mat chemical" from their bread following a petition I started.[1] Kraft decided to remove artificial food dyes from their kids' mac and cheese products after I stormed their headquarters with over 200,000 petitions.[2] Chick-fil-A's chicken went antibiotic free following my meetings with them urging them to do so.[3] Anheuser-Busch and Miller-Coors both agreed to publish their ingredients for the first time in history following another of my petitions.[4] I was finishing up my first book, exposing the chemicals in our food, and it was slated to be out in a few short months. I had just published an investigation into Starbucks' famous Pumpkin Spice Latte,[5] calling them out for their use of "class IV" caramel coloring (a chemical linked to cancer).[6] This piece went viral, with millions of views and shares (which ultimately led to Starbucks dropping this coloring from their drinks).[7] We were really shaking up the food world. Needless to say, the industry was not happy. Changing their products meant losing money. And they were scrambling to stop our momentum.

Although it was a very exciting time, I was quite nervous going into this interview. Our success in getting billion-dollar food companies to change was leading to some serious blowback. There were articles coming out calling me a fearmonger and worse. While I knew that many of my critics had an agenda—they were working with the very companies I was criticizing—I was cautiously optimistic that the *Times* would take a different approach.

That said, I spent countless hours preparing for the interview. I underwent a mock grilling by my book publicist. We sat in the hotel restaurant for a couple of hours leading up to the interview to make sure I could handle any question thrown my way. After this prep I thought I was ready, so I went upstairs and thought about what to wear to the interview. I ended up wearing my favorite staples: a cozy sweater with a big heart on it and a pair of heart-shaped sparkly earrings. We decided to meet at one of my favorite organic restaurants in New York City, a place called ABC Kitchen. The restaurant is magical. The windows and decor are all white or soft pink, almost heavenlike, and the food features lots of vegetables prepared beautifully. I walked in a few minutes early and the *Times* reporter walked in right behind me. We locked eyes and I said hello with a smile. But she didn't smile back, nor did she ask how I was doing. As a Southerner, I'm used to warmer greetings and a little small talk about the weather. Her coldness threw me completely off; it was like she sucked the air right out of the room. When we sat down at the table, I tried to lighten up the mood and started talking about the menu. I was excited to order my favorite dish—squash toast—but the reporter quickly dismissed it, lamenting that she didn't eat gluten.

She turned on the tape recorder and we began the interview. It went on for an hour and a half. I literally did not look up from the table. It was like the entire bustling restaurant had disappeared around me. When she got to the question I'd been waiting for, asking why so many scientists were against my work and advocacy, I gave her my most honest answer. Many of these scientists, I said, are working for the food lobby—they have a strong financial incentive to keep the status quo. Some are paid directly by the companies, or get grants from them, while others are supported by front groups. She insisted I was wrong, telling me that these were independent experts. Although she didn't mention any of my critics by name, I had a pretty good idea who she was talking about because I'd already been attacked by them in several media outlets.

I left that interview and headed straight to the airport. I called my husband from the car. When he asked "How did it go?" I responded, "Dicey—it's probably going to be another hit piece," bracing myself for another highly critical article featuring food industry scientists claiming I was a misinformed woman needlessly worried about harmless chemicals.

While we were waiting for the article to be published, my first book, *The Food Babe Way*, came out. The book was a huge success, hitting the *New York Times* bestseller list, remaining there for months. I was thrilled that so many people were interested in our movement and learning the truth about our food.

Eventually, the *Times* published their article.[8] They described me as "Public Enemy No. 1 of big food companies" (which I actually found quite flattering), but as expected, the rest of the piece weighed heavily on criticisms of my work. The reporter cited four different experts as critics of mine. Although she told me these experts were independent, only one of them was an actual food scientist.[9] And the fact that this scientist sat on the board of directors of Sensient Technologies Corporation,[10] the largest manufacturer of caramel color,[11] was absurdly left out of the article. This is the very same color I was actively campaigning to get out of Starbucks at the time. Corporate records reflect that this scientist, Dr. Fergus Clydesdale, was getting over $100,000 in annual compensation from the caramel coloring industry.[12] The fact that Dr. Clydesdale served on various committees for food industry trade[13] and front groups[14] was also not mentioned. In this book, we will further explore the ties between experts and the industry, and how they are slyly using the media to further their agenda.

You see, mouthpieces of the food and chemical industries have been fooling reporters for years. In this case, rather than investigate the dangerous ingredients in countless foods, they focused on me as a messenger of change, and questioned what right I had to speak out about what I've learned. Instead, shouldn't the media question why certain scientists and doctors are defending a food system that is clearly making us sick?

Months later, I obtained some internal e-mails via a Freedom of Information Act (FOIA) request, which included an e-mail from *The New York Times* reporter to one of my critics quoted in her article about me. "I'm already getting complaints I wasn't hard enough on her," she said. I've since discovered this particular critic, Dr. Joe Schwarcz, has received speaking fee payments from the agrochemical industry (Bayer CropScience, Monsanto, and Croplife Canada, to name a few[15]). In one 2014 e-mail he asked a CropLife Canada representative, "Let me be mercenary . . . what is the arrangement there?" upon being asked to speak at an upcoming event that CropLife was arranging at Algonquin College. "What is the financial arrangement?" Schwarcz went on to clarify, as CropLife readily assured him, "CropLife Canada will pay your travel and speaking fee; Algonquin College will provide the space and invite who they would like to attend." Schwarcz spoke on April 3, 2014. Advertisements[16] for the event touted Schwarcz as "one of Canada's foremost science experts, as he speaks about the nutritional value of organic food versus conventional foods, genetically modified foods, and debunk some common myths about food in Canada and the science behind it." Missing from this promotional material was any mention that his talk was being funded by the agrichemical industry. And in another e-mail he revealed how much he relished the opportunity to take part in the *Times* piece, telling the reporter, "It's always fun to do a little Babe bashing. Such an easy target."[17] As expected, the attacks in the media continued and got even more vicious.

They wanted to shut me up. I'm a tough woman, and I can take my fair share of criticism. But what I refuse to accept is an environment that propagates lies and perpetuates ignorance among the public about what we should eat. We all have the right to learn about our food and what's in it, and to demand transparency from the companies who are selling us these products.

From the very start, my mission has been simple: I want to tell people the truth about the food they're eating. My advocacy is why companies like Subway, General Mills, Starbucks, Kraft, and Anheuser-Busch have had to either change their ingredients or become more transparent. They're not doing this because they want to, or because they finally feel bad about selling us processed food full of artificial crap. They're doing it because we made them do it, because we finally insisted that it's not okay to sell us stuff that makes us sick.

And we've made progress, lots of progress. When you walk around a supermarket these days, it's clear that the major trends are toward food that is organic, natural, and healthy. These trends aren't an accident. They exist because we've taught people about the dangers of food that's loaded up with dyes, weed killer, fake sugars, artificial flavors, and countless other additives that have no business being in our kitchen. Unfortunately, the food industry is the one with the deep pockets. They have the means to keep marketing their lies, pushing their products, and attacking critics of the industry like myself.

I wrote this book because it was time to fight back. It wasn't enough to tell people about the ingredients that were making them sick—if I was going to help fix the system, I also needed to expose the lies that kept the status quo in place. I needed to give people the ability to see through these lies so they can make informed choices about the food they are eating and feeding to their families.

This book is inspired by people like you, people who are trying to take the best care of themselves and become informed about the food we eat. While the *Times* piece hit me really hard, I was lucky enough to spend the next several months traveling around the country on my book tour. I met thousands of readers—together, we are known as the Food Babe Army—and made some of the most meaningful connections of my life. I heard stories of healing families and children and how changing your diet can help change your life.

And that's when I decided that I wasn't going to let the critics beat me down. Not when many of them are cashing checks from the Big Food or Chemical industry. Not when they're telling lies. So I turned off my Google News alerts. I got a Facebook moderator and stopped reading those hateful comments and tweets. I focused on what matters, which is this powerful sense of purpose I feel when educating people about how to eat food that makes us feel good.

One of my favorite sayings goes like this: "No mud, no lotus." What the saying means is that without struggle there is no progress. Together, we've struggled through all the food industry's lies. We've put up with their terrible products and dealt with the downward spiral of obesity, diabetes and disease they've largely caused.

And now we have a chance to finally change things. But first we have to understand who and what we're fighting against.

We have to understand the lies so we can learn the truth about our food.

Who is doing the lying?

The food industry, that's who.

Remember how the tobacco industry lied to us about the dangers of cigarettes? Or how the drug companies have hidden information about the dangerous side effects of their medicines? Well, the same untruths, cover-ups, and deceptive practices are occurring in the food industry.

Many so-called "healthy foods" are not healthy at all.

Many food products are not what their labels say they are.

Many studies on foods are being manipulated, and are funded by self-serving food companies.

Many statistics are being taken out of context, with deliberate attempts to mislead.

Many medical groups, doctors, dietitians, and other health experts are taking money in exchange for endorsements, regardless of whether or not a food or food product is healthy.

It's shameless.

You just need to take a short step back in history to see how the Big Food industry corrupts everything it touches. In the mid-1930s, Margaret Rudkin began baking loaves of stone-ground whole-wheat bread to help her son Mark, who had severe food allergies and asthma that prevented him from eating processed foods. This bread was quite different from the mass-produced fluffy white breads that proliferated at the time. Her first loaf was not a success: it was "hard as a rock," she said, and didn't rise at all. But Margaret kept at it and by 1937 she was selling her healthy loaves (made with real butter and honey) to the local market, which her family claimed was the best tasting bread they'd ever had. She named her bread after her small farm in Fairfield, Connecticut: Pepperidge Farm.[18]

Before long, her bread gained a devoted following. Doctors recommended it to patients with digestive issues; newspapers celebrated it as a "healthful bread" eaten by America's "elite"; Margaret was able to charge more than twice as much as ordinary commercially baked white loaves cost because her bread came with added health benefits.

As the years passed, Margaret slowly increased the product line of Pepperidge Farm. One of her biggest hits was a fish-shaped cracker she discovered while traveling in Europe. The original recipe was simple, consisting of little more than wheat flour, nonfat milk, yeast, leavening, salt, and spices. As snacks go, it was a fine alternative since it didn't contain any preservatives or artificial flavors or colors.

In 1961, Pepperidge Farm was bought by Campbell's Soup Company. It was an early example of food industry consolidation. While Campbell's initially made few changes to Pepperidge Farm's lineup, by the 1970s they began introducing new products and revising the recipes for old ones in ways that dramatically differed from Margaret's original mission.

Consider the cake that my family ate to celebrate countless birthdays: Pepperidge Farm Golden Layer Cake. It came out of the freezer section in a white box. I remember struggling to wait while it thawed on the counter. I always begged for a second piece.

My family didn't know it at the time, but we were being duped. My unsuspecting parents probably thought the cake was frozen because it had been baked fresh (probably on a farm as the label suggested) and needed to be preserved. They had no idea that it was actually preserved not by freezing but by a slew of additives and other artificial ingredients that kept it from breaking down. The ingredients of this cake are like a greatest hits of food ingredients to avoid. The first ingredient is sugar (of course), followed by ingredients like hydrogenated oils, high-fructose corn syrup, regular corn syrup, mono- and diglycerides, and polysorbate 60. In this book, you'll come to understand why many of these ingredients are potentially dangerous.

And it's not just the Golden Layer Cake. A quick glance at the Pepperidge Farm product line reveals many of the fundamental problems with processed food. Those goldfish crackers, for instance, now come in dozens of different flavors, many of which are laced with hidden MSG additives. Some Pepperidge Farm breads, meanwhile, are filled with the artificial sweetener sucralose, chemically refined soybean oil, and diacetyl tartaric acid esters of mono- and diglycerides (DATEM). I doubt Margaret Rudkin would approve.

Of course, Pepperidge Farm isn't unique. Most of the frozen cakes, snack foods, and breads in the supermarket are just as bad. But I'm picking on Pepperidge Farm because the company had such virtuous origins. As such, it perfectly illustrates how Big Food corrupts our food system, selling us lies so we keep buying its products even when they make us sick. We see that Pepperidge Farm logo with the red barn and we think it must be wholesome and natural, just like the first healthy breads sold by Margaret Rudkin. But the logo at this point is just meaningless marketing: many of these products are industrialized foods, full of ingredients made in chemistry labs and giant factories. They are crammed full of salt, sugar, and concentrated flavorings so we can't stop eating them. While Margaret Rudkin set out to create a bread that helped her son feel better, most of these products are designed solely to pad the profit margins of Big Food, even if it means we might get sick.

For way too long, we've outsourced our dietary decisions to Big Food, letting them decide what we put in our bodies. We eat their sugary cereals for breakfast and their frozen cakes for dessert; we make sandwiches full of their processed bread, processed meats, and mass-produced cheeses; we gulp their sodas and then, when we're trying to lose weight, switch to their diet sodas, which are just as bad, if not worse! This is a huge mistake because Big Food doesn't seem to put our health first— they just care about their bottom line. And that's why we can't rely on them for our meals, snacks, or food advice. In this book, you'll learn how to see through their lies and make food choices that are good for your health.

■ ■ ■

My name is Vani Hari, aka the Food Babe, and I'm one of the country's leading food activists and bloggers. What exactly does that mean? Well, I—along with my Food Babe Army of fellow activists—campaign food companies to persuade them to remove unhealthy additives or to disclose the ingredients in their products. As a result of our efforts, Kraft dropped the artificial dyes (Yellow #5 and Yellow #6) from all of its Mac & Cheese products. After Kraft's announcement, other major food conglomerates, like General Mills, Mars, Hershey's, Nestlé, and Kellogg's, vowed to be artificial color–free in coming years. Subway eliminated the risky dough conditioner azodicarbonamide from its bread after our petition[19] and now most major brands have followed suit. General Mills is dumping the controversial preservative BHT from cereals, just as it did overseas.[20] Panera Bread got rid of 150 artificial additives from its products, and those additives included artificial colors, BHT, nitrates, high-fructose corn syrup, hidden MSG, and partially hydrogenated oils.[21] Chipotle officially did away with all genetically modified (GMO) ingredients in its food (excluding animal products and drinks).[22] This is just a handful of the changes we have helped create.

In fact, even Pepperidge Farm has begun to change. Campbell's, their parent company, announced that they are switching to antibiotic-free chicken, eliminating BPA from cans, cutting out all artificial colors and flavors,[23] and leaving the biggest food industry lobbying group. After Campbell's announced they would begin labeling GMO ingredients, including on Pepperidge Farm products, I organized a letter-writing campaign thanking the former CEO of Campbell's, Denise Morrison, for taking that important step. Denise then sent me a picture on Twitter of all the letters on her desk. Eventually Denise resigned as CEO because even these positive changes could not change the trajectory of the shifting food economy. Campbell's has continued to see declining sales for their processed food lines.

The moral here is that change is hard, but it's possible. In just a few years, we've helped eliminate lots of bad and dangerous ingredients from products eaten billions of times every year. When we work together, we can make sure our voices are heard.

Because of these successes, *Time* magazine described me as one of the 30 Most Influential People on the Internet,[24] and The Daily Meal called me one of the 13 Most Powerful Women in Food.[25] It's nice to be recognized, but it has cost me.

I've been in the hot seat as well as in the spotlight since starting my blog in 2011. I've been falsely accused of demonizing common food ingredients, pushing alternatives for profit, and declaring victory when a big company makes positive changes in its product. All of this is untrue—except the latter. I love declaring victory every time food companies change their ingredients.

Yes, there has been tremendous blowback to what I do. There are those unfair articles in places like the *Times*, of course, and I'm also personally subjected to hate speech, harassment, and cyberbullying on a daily basis. Instead of focusing on the issues I've raised about the food industry, they attack me as a woman, often in ways they'd never attack a man. Death threats, rape threats, drive-bys of my home, all to intimidate me and get me to stop.

Although I don't have evidence pointing to one specific company, group, or individual who was involved, these terrifying threats escalated to the point where I had to ban numerous profiles from my Facebook page who have been persuaded (and in some instances paid) by the public relations departments of the food companies to harass me on a daily basis. Some of these "Internet trolls," as they've been termed, include top executives from the largest food companies and scientist professors from public universities, who have also been given a platform in the media. Rick Berman—a controversial PR agent who has been described by some as "Dr. Evil"—called me a "food bimbo" in the *Washington Times*.[26] But I refuse to stop. My life's mission is to help people like you live healthier, better lives, regardless of food industry influences.

I feel so strongly about the truth about our food because I wasn't always the healthy person I am today. For most of my life, I ate terribly. I was a candy addict, drank soda, never ate green vegetables, frequented fast food restaurants, and gorged on processed food (we all have our moments!). My diet landed me where a bad diet typically does: in a hospital bed. There I was at the age of 22, feeling weak and fragile instead of strong and healthy. It was then that I decided to make health my number-one priority.

I used my newfound inspiration for living a healthy life to investigate what is really in our food, how it's grown, and what chemicals are used in its production. I didn't go to nutrition school to learn this. I had to teach myself everything, and I spent thousands of hours researching and talking to experts. As I began to learn more, I could see through big business marketing tactics and lengthy food labels. Most importantly, the more I learned and the more lessons I put into action, the better I felt—and I wanted to tell everyone about it!

Personal attacks and threats don't scare me in the least anymore; they come with the territory. I hope the trolls know that I will not stop. I will not shut up. I will not fade away. I am a very vocal, widely followed consumer advocate on a lifelong mission to educate the public about what is really happening to our food, and how we have been misled by the food industry, paid media messengers, and slick, slimy con artists operating under the guise of being "independent" experts.

Being lied to is just wrong.

It's time to learn the truth.

TIRED OF BEING FED LIES?

This is a new kind of diet and health book. I provide you with the knowledge you need to make informed decisions. I help you overcome the obstacles standing in the way of your taking greater responsibility for your health. I help you dig deeper and look for your own evidence of deception in today's food world. I help you take control of your life—and change it for the better.

This book isn't only a manifesto that recounts the sins of the food industry. I go beyond that. I give you recommendations for personal action that can protect you from cheap, processed, unhealthy foods and the health problems and suffering they cause. In every chapter, I offer action steps—including my 48-Hour Toxin Takedown at the end of the book—that will help you avoid chemical onslaughts from food, and get healthy in the process. You'll end your sugar and processed food addictions, lose pound after pound, never diet again, and rejuvenate your energy levels, mental fitness, and overall well-being.

Health is the greatest gift for a happy, productive life and the greatest wealth anyone can have, but we could lose it at any moment if we're not vigilant. All it really takes is the belief that you are worth the effort. I invite you to step up, take charge, claim that gift, and keep it forever.

Now is the best time to change your life.

Vani Hari

Part I

THE LIARS

CHAPTER 1

The Guilty Parties:
Lies and Ties

I crossed paths recently with an old food friend: Fig Newtons. When I was growing up, these cookies were a staple in the cupboard and in my lunchbox. This newer version, I noticed, claimed to be 100 percent whole grain, made with real fruit. Sounds healthy, right?

I read labels like they're bestsellers, so when I took a closer look at the list of ingredients in this cookie, my jaw dropped. I couldn't believe how many processed chemicals they contained. There was sugar under at least three different names, and artificial flavorings.

Ironically, these popular cookies were created back in the 19th century as a health food. Physicians believed that a daily intake of biscuits and fruit would cure digestive problems. This advice inspired a baker in Philadelphia, who invented a novel machine that would wrap pastry dough around fig paste, to make an enchanting little cookie. His recipe was purchased by a larger Massachusetts bakery, and the product was named after the town of Newton, Massachusetts. The Fig Newton was born in 1891.[1]

Fast forward to the present: Fig Newtons are a perfect example of how chemicals are replacing nutrients in the foods we eat. They contain some of the basic ingredients we'd use to bake our own cookies, like flour, sugar, and baking soda, but most of the ingredients are not what you'd find in your pantry. (Many of them can't even be purchased in a grocery store.) Here's a sampling:

There are three types of added sugar in Nabisco's 100% Whole Grain Wheat Triple Berry Newtons: regular sugar, corn syrup, and invert sugar. All of which are refined sugars—and scarily associated with obesity, heart disease, cancer, dementia, and liver damage. You'll eat 12 grams of sugar (3 teaspoons) in just two small Fig Newtons. And how many of us can stop at just two cookies?

Fat is a chief ingredient and shows up in the form of canola oil, a heavily refined oil that goes through an insane amount of processing with chemical solvents (like hexane, a neurotoxin[2]), steamers, neutralizers, de-waxers, bleach, and deodorizers.[3] Although it does indeed contain real fruit, these little Triple Berry Newtons are still artificially flavored and dyed with Red 40, a risky dye that requires a warning label in Europe.[4] These flavors and dyes have zero nutritional value and are solely used by the industry to mimic the look and taste of real food with fake chemicals.

I'm not picking on Fig Newtons. (Well, maybe just a little.) But I could have just as easily chosen any one of the thousands of brands of processed foods on supermarket shelves these days. I'm just calling out these cookies because they market themselves as a healthier alternative. Yet some versions of Fig Newtons are still laced with refined sugar, refined flour, preservatives, synthetic food dyes, and artificial flavors. If Fig Newtons are this bad, just imagine what an "unhealthy" cookie is like.

Fig Newtons are an example of the Big Food industry at work. These multinational companies are really good at selling us fake food, produced in giant factories from a long list of already highly processed ingredients. They sell us these products because they are highly profitable, even if it means we're consuming dangerous chemicals, additives, and toxic ingredients.

And it gets worse than that. It's intentional. Food companies have big R&D departments for this very reason—to make their food *addictive*.[5] If it wasn't, they'd have a much harder time staying in business. As a result, American families are compelled to keep gobbling down loads of processed foods, full of way too much sugar and risky additives . . . fake food. It's no surprise that this has led to escalating rates of obesity, diabetes, and other chronic diseases. But we believe we need processed food—because we've been conditioned to crave it. The big companies rake in the profits; we pay with our health.

We've been processing food since the dawn of time, initially for good reasons. Cooking, fermenting, canning, freezing, and other preservation methods are forms of processing, and they have generally created safer foods.

In recent decades, however, Big Food has taken processing to an entirely new level, creating franken "foods" that are bad for us but good for their bottom line. However, before I explain everything that's wrong with these food products—and how we can learn to eat better—we need to understand how we got here, scarfing down processed industrial foods that are full of crap you'd never want to feed yourself or your family.

It's a sordid tale.

BIG FOOD'S DIRTY SECRET

When you sell food that makes people sick, it turns out you have to spend a lot of time and money trying to convince people it's not your fault. Just as the tobacco industry invested millions of dollars trying (in vain) to discredit the research showing the link between smoking and lung cancer, so has Big Food invested huge resources into persuading people that their unhealthy products aren't behind the obesity, type 2 diabetes, and chronic diseases affecting Americans on a grand scale.

One of the main ways the food industry does this is by creating entities known as "front groups" whose purpose is to spread information that is favorable to the industry, all while hiding the fact that they're working for the food and chemical industries. These organizations have names that sound grassroots, but they're actually paid for and organized by giant corporations with deep pockets. These front groups advance their claims that processed foods full of artificial additives, factory farmed meat, and GMOs are safe, wholesome, and beyond reproach.

In many instances, Big Food and Chemical companies will try to hide their ties to a front group.[6] Here's a typical sequence of events:

A large corporation donates money to a foundation or charity that gives the appearance of being independent but acts as a funnel for the corporation's money going forward.

This foundation funds a new organization to be established to "communicate" to the public. Sometimes, a PR firm is hired to create this organization. They may even create multiple organizations down the line to further hide their connections to industry. These are all front groups.

This new front group creates a respectable-looking website and establishes social media accounts, stating that its mission is to spread the truth about science and food.

The front group creates "experts" in the field by training farmers, dietitians, bloggers, and scientists how to help spread their messages about the "safety" of GMOs, food additives, factory farming practices, or pesticides. These experts may be paid or given other accommodations to do this work for the front group organization. If they are moms, this is considered a bonus, because the industry knows that moms typically make household food decisions and will be more widely accepted by the public.[7]

The organization will then recommend these trained experts to journalists who are writing for major media publications. You'll often see these front groups and their trained messengers quoted in the media without any mention of their connections to the industries they work for, and without any conflict-of-interest disclaimers.

In many instances, these trained farmers, scientists, and "mommy bloggers" will also write their own blogs or pen articles for bigger mainstream publications. Likewise, they create

Facebook groups and pages that will be used to poke fun at activists (like me) and try to disrupt the work we are doing. This process has been duplicated dozens of times and will continue as long as they are not exposed.

An investigation by Friends of the Earth documented the sheer scale of these propaganda efforts. They found, for instance, that four of the largest food and chemical trade associations spent over $500 million from 2009 to 2013 on these efforts. They also uncovered that 14 of the largest front groups working for the food industry spent about $126 million during that same time period, often without fully disclosing where their funding came from.[8]

FRONT GROUPS: WHO ARE THEY?

A good example of a prominent front group[9] is the American Council on Science and Health (ACSH). According to documents leaked to the publication *Mother Jones*, this self-proclaimed "pro-science consumer advocacy organization" has received significant funding from a who's who list of Big Food and chemical companies, such as Bayer, McDonald's, Coca-Cola, and Monsanto.[10]

ACSH continues to dispute any ties to the food and chemical industry, stating:

> We are not a trade association, we do not represent any industry, we were created to be the science alternative to 'news' that is often little more than hype based on exaggerated findings, and to help policymakers see past scaremongers, activist groups who have targeted GMOs, vaccines, conventional agriculture, nuclear power, natural gas, and 'chemicals,' while peddling health scares and fad diets. The Council's primary aim is to inform the public and policymakers of good science while debunking the junk.[11]

Color me skeptical: I sincerely doubt that these big companies are spending millions of dollars on a group without influencing their findings and positions. (And isn't it strange that their positions are always pro-industry?) Nonetheless, major media outlets such as *USA Today* regularly publish columns written by ACSH's president and a senior fellow, without any mention of their apparent ties to corporate interests.[12]

Now consider the Cornell Alliance for Science, housed at Cornell University. This prestigious-sounding group just happens to be the public relations arm for the agrochemical industry.[13] Its stance is squarely pro-GMO and pro-chemical.[14]

The Cornell Alliance for Science claims to have zero industry ties, yet their partners have included several organizations funded by biotechnology companies who sell GMOs and the chemicals used in conjunction with them. To muddle industry ties, they no longer publish a list of "Partners" on their website; however, Internet archives[15] reveal that one partner has been the International Service for the Acquisition of Agri-biotech Applications, which receives funding from Monsanto (maker of GMO seeds) and CropLife, a trade organization for Monsanto and other biotech giants.[16] See how they try to obscure affiliations like these?

The group got called out by 67 farmers who sent a letter to Cornell, urging them to evict the Cornell Alliance for Science for their biased stance on GMOs. "Nothing in the materials or programs of 'The Alliance for Science' is anything but entirely pro-biotechnology. They are without balance or significant critical evaluation of the range of agricultural systems and technologies that exist in food production today," wrote Elizabeth Henderson, an organic farmer from Wayne County, New York.[17]

Meanwhile, the Cornell Alliance for Science provides leadership training to students, farmers, and scientists, many of whom have a background in marketing, business, or journalism, so they are better prepared to use their communication skills to promote the use of GMOs, along with chemical-intrusive agriculture, and to slam activists who are fighting for more sustainable practices. It also offers journalism fellowships with cash awards for "in-depth reporting on important topics in agriculture related to food security and innovative agricultural practices" (in other words, GMOs and pesticides).[18] They put on a front that they are activists trying to help farmers when they are actually just conducting PR work for the biotech industry. It's appalling.

Another example of an industry front group is the Center for Food Integrity (CFI). Its members include trade groups like the National Restaurant Association, the Grocery Manufacturers Association, the American Farm Bureau Federation, the Dairy Farmers of America, and companies like Monsanto and Hershey's,[19] with a primary mission to downplay any public concerns about chemical food additives. They spent a whopping $23,225,098 between 2012 and 2016 on marketing and publicity efforts pushing the agenda of their members.[20] It might not surprise you to learn that I've personally been a frequent target of CFI's media attacks, especially since I've persuaded numerous CFI members (past and present, such as Chick-fil-A) to remove additives from their food and adopt antibiotic-free policies in the sourcing of their meat.

Then there's the U.S. Farmers and Ranchers Alliance (USFRA), a front group partnered with biotech and chemical giants like Bayer and Monsanto, along with Elanco (makers of conventional animal feed) and Merck Animal Health (makers of animal antibiotics and vaccines).[21] USFRA spends millions every year promoting the use of routine antibiotics in farm animals, GMOs, and the safety of synthetic pesticides and conventional agriculture.[22] They have reportedly trained thousands of farmers and ranchers throughout the U.S. to be spokespeople promoting these dangerous aims, teaching them how to use USFRA talking points.[23]

In 2016 USFRA launched a campaign called "Straight Talk," hoping to dissuade companies from removing GMOs from their food products. The launch came shortly after Dannon pledged that it would eliminate GMO feed from some of the animals that produce its dairy products (a giant blow to the GMO industry since GMOs are most widely used to feed farm animals). The industry paper *Agri-Pulse* reported, "USFRA CEO Randy Krotz didn't go into specifics on which companies will be approached through the campaign, but there is a list of 'a dozen food companies that we are very, very focused on' and that 'the list would not surprise you at all.'"[24]

TRADE GROUPS

Similar to front groups are "trade groups" or "trade associations." These are organizations openly funded by businesses that operate in order to promote their interests. They participate in activities such as lobbying, political donations, advertising, education, and publishing. Every business and industry has them—and Big Food is no different. Examples include the Calorie Control Council representing low-calorie sweetener manufacturers, the Sugar Association representing sugar growers, the American Beverage Association representing bottled beverage and soda makers, and the Grocery Manufacturers Association representing packaged food and beverage companies. Besides lobbying, trade groups frequently funnel their money to front groups to further their message to the public. These trade groups play a significant role in shaping public opinion about food and beverages, and they have a far-ranging influence on food policies. Their influence on the American diet cannot be overstated.

Government agencies, namely the U.S. departments of Agriculture and Health and Human Services, develop the U.S. Dietary Guidelines for Americans, and they take recommendations from various groups, including trade associations.

According to an investigation into trade groups by the Center for Public Integrity, "Big spenders included the American Beverage Association, which has been shelling out millions to try and keep cities and states from taxing sugary drinks." Yet, they found most of the money spent by trade groups goes toward efforts to influence the public. "They certainly want to influence the general public, because the general public will then influence the politicians, the lawmakers or the regulators in that particular industry," said Steve Barrett, editor-in-chief of *PRWeek*, in referencing their investigation.[25]

This type of influence peddling by front groups and trade associations goes on all the time. It is their main reason for being.

Worst of all, it works.

BIG FOOD AND ACADEMICS

Who do you trust for information about your food? Do you trust the government? How about food companies themselves? Most people would say "no way!" to both those questions. The industry has found that the public generally doesn't trust information coming directly from them, so they deploy a stealthy tactic. You see, the public is often trusting of information that comes from credentialed experts who appear to be completely independent and separate from industry, such as academics at publicly funded universities. That's why Big Food and Chemical regularly work with university scientists behind closed doors to spread misinformation about food and nutrition, dispute activists, repeat industry talking points, and generally manipulate the public. They essentially use certain university professors as puppets to advance their message. In general, they do this under the name of "science outreach" or "science communication," but when it is propagated by industry it is really just industry propaganda with a fancy name slapped on it. It's more about protecting the bottom line of the industry than actually spreading the truth about science.

I've known about this connection between academics and industry for a long time, and have had personal experience with it. Let me give you one telling example.

Soon after the Food Babe Army petitioned Kraft and Subway to change their ingredients, a professor from the University of Florida, Dr. Kevin M. Folta, appeared on the scene and began criticizing our work (and me personally). This particular professor is a very vocal proponent of GMO technology and the chemicals used along with them made by Monsanto (he even reportedly drank Roundup weed killer mixed with Diet Mountain Dew at some of his talks to demonstrate its safety).[26] He also explicitly stated on several occasions that he was an independent public scientist with no relationship to Monsanto.[27] Thus, he was trusted by many.

Folta ramped up his attacks against me after I was invited to his campus to give a talk for the university's Common Reading Program, nominated by one of the staff members: "We admire your work and believe that our students would greatly benefit from hearing you speak," they wrote. During the talk to hundreds of freshman, I discussed my journey as a food activist, including the campaigns I had led to get the food industry to change by removing controversial chemicals and improving their food practices. The students were required to read *The Good Food Revolution* by Will Allen in preparation for my talk, so they were primed to hear more about the central theme of an unjust food system that produces unhealthy food for the majority. After my talk, I stuck around for an hour or so and met candidly with many of the students and some teachers who attended. Folta was in the auditorium but did not approach me or come up to meet me like so many others did.

I later discovered that Folta e-mailed his boss the morning after my talk, writing, "Over an hour of bad science, lies about food and farming, poisoning the minds of about 500 UF undergrads. No Q&A session. Now we have to fix it."[28] He proceeded to write on his blog, "There's something that dies inside when you are a faculty member that works hard to teach about food, farming and science, and your own university brings in a crackpot to unravel all of the information you have brought to students . . . If this is a charismatic leader of a new food movement it is quite a disaster. She's uninformed, uneducated, trite and illogical. She's afraid of science and intellectual engagement. She's Oz candy at best."[29]

Needless to say, Monsanto was pleased that Folta attended my talk and wrote a discrediting piece about me on his blog. Monsanto executive Lisa Drake e-mailed Folta a couple days later: "Just saw this post—you rock! Glad you were able to stop by, but a sacrifice for sure. Lisa."[30] Folta also got praise from public relations firm Look East (formerly CMA), which has worked with Monsanto: "I found your piece on Food Babe's visit to your campus extremely entertaining. Nice work."[31] The president and CEO of the American Seed Trade Association (a Big Ag trade group) wrote him privately as well: "I've been following your work, statements, speeches on science v. advocacy and I want to say thank you. Your willingness to standup to the likes of the 'Food Babe' and call BS is wonderful and you do it in such an graceful manner."[32]

He didn't stop there. Folta closely followed our work for months following my visit to UF. Every time we made headway on an important issue, Dr. Folta, who as I mentioned, called himself an independent public scientist, was there to refute our claims and throw in some ad hominem attacks in the media. Here are a couple direct quotes from the news:

"The fact that she is able to mobilize this army of blind followers who reject science and follow her words, to smear and harm the reputations of companies that are doing nothing wrong."—*The Atlantic*, 2/11/2015.[33]

"Kevin M. Folta, the chairman of the horticultural sciences department at the University of Florida, described Ms. Hari's lecture at the university last October as a 'corrupt message of bogus science and abject food terrorism.'"—*The New York Times*, 3/15/2015.[34]

Folta even e-mailed Adam Carolla's office on three occasions, hoping to get on his popular podcast. "I'm a huge fan of the podcast. I'm also a professor that leads one of the USA's leading ag programs at a huge university. I know a ton about farming, food, GMO, food terrorism (like the Food Babe and other morons that want to scare people out of eating), food allergies, and food's interface with contemporary society."[35]

My intuition and common sense told me there was no way this guy would be engaging in personal attacks like this unless he was in cahoots with Big Food or chemical companies, but he kept denying any alliances or funding arrangements. He maintained that he was an independent public scientist working for the University of Florida. As a result, the media portrayed him as an unbiased scientist and he was continually given a platform to bash me publicly.

Then came a bombshell report published in *The New York Times* several months later. When I saw this story on the front page of the paper, my jaw dropped wide open. The piece, entitled "Food Industry Enlisted Academics in G.M.O. Lobbying War, Emails Show," described how the chemical and food industries work with public university scientists to advance their agendas to consumers.[36] They published hundreds of private e-mails between Dr. Folta, Monsanto, front groups, and the public relations firm Ketchum. (The e-mails came to light after Freedom of Information Act requests were submitted by the nonprofit group U.S. Right to Know.[37]) The vast series of e-mails indicate that although Folta repeatedly denied having any connection to Monsanto, he solicited a $25,000 grant from the company to further his biotech communications efforts; the money was paid to the University of Florida. (In an e-mail to Monsanto executives, he promised "a solid return on the investment.") This is a clear conflict of interest and contrary to his previous claims that he has no ties to Monsanto. As was reported in the *Gainesville Sun*, after this information went public, Folta tried to give Monsanto a refund: "I talked to Monsanto about returning the money. They are totally against it, said it looks like an admission of guilt." Monsanto's spokesperson told the paper, "We funded Dr. Folta's proposal through an unrestricted grant to the University of Florida with no strings attached—which means we cannot make any formal requirements on how the funds are used."[38] The university later made amends by reallocating the funds to benefit a food pantry.

SCIENCE FOR SALE

Sadly, these conflicts go on all the time. You run into them constantly with scientific studies about nutrition, particularly in studies of beverages. According to a 2007 report in *PLOS Medicine*, research results appear to be biased in favor of the food manufacturers who pay for the studies.[39] The numbers are staggering: research funded solely by the beverage industry was four to eight times more likely to draw conclusions favorable to industry sponsors than were studies with no industry funding. Dr. David Ludwig, the study's senior author, noted that not only do such findings attract frequent media attention, but they also influence governmental and professional dietary guidelines, as well as Food and Drug Administration (FDA) decisions on health claims allowed on foods and beverages. Sadly, when it comes to scientific research, Big Food is essentially able to buy the results it wants. At the very least, such biased data confuses consumers, obscuring the truth so we keep on buying their processed junk.

Marion Nestle, a nutrition professor and author, summed this up beautifully in an interview with the American Association of University Professors:

> Sponsorship almost invariably predicts the results of research . . . results are highly likely to favor the sponsor's interest. The companies are not buying the results, although it sometimes seems that way. Instead, it seems to me that researchers who are willing to accept grants from food companies tend to be less critical about the way they design their studies. I often notice that sponsored studies lack appropriately rigorous controls. One way to understand this is to suggest that scientists who accept corporate sponsorship have internalized the values of the sponsor so thoroughly that they think themselves independent . . . As a rule, corporate funding discourages critical thinking—or promotes uncritical thinking—about the importance of individual foods or nutrients in healthful diets. Sponsored studies have only one purpose—to establish a basis for marketing claims. They are not carried out to promote public health.[40]

Boom.

But wait: there's more. According to a report titled "Nutrition Scientists on the Take from Big Food," authored by attorney and food advocate Michele Simon, an alarming number of studies on nutrition are corrupted by groups and companies connected to Big Food.[41] Her fascinating report details how these companies control and influence the science surrounding nutritional research. Also included in the report is an expose of the American Society of Nutrition (ASN), which is considered a renowned academic organization specializing in nutrition research. In reality, the ASN is sponsored by a gaggle of industry conglomerates like Cargill, Coca-Cola, Kellogg's, PepsiCo, and McDonald's (who have each paid at least $10,000 per year for the spot). Meanwhile, the ASN publishes the *American Journal of Clinical Nutrition* (*AJCN*), considered one of the most respected scientific journals in the field of nutrition. Dubiously, though, at least one researcher in cahoots with Big Food serves on the AJCN's editorial board, which determines what gets published in the journal.

Worth mentioning too is that the AJCN contends that processed foods are not the enemy and promotes the idea that nearly every food is processed, since processing also refers to food that is cut, frozen, or cooked. That's a weak argument, if you ask me. I think there's a huge difference between a bag of frozen peas and a bag of Doritos.

To further complicate matters, industry-funded influence is not always disclosed in published research papers. A *Journal of Public Health Policy* paper found that although several studies funded by Coca-Cola reported "no influence by the funder, the correspondence describes detailed exchanges on the study design, presentation of results and acknowledgement of funding. This raises important questions about the meaning of standard statements on conflicts of interest."[42] This allows food companies like Coca-Cola to influence public policy and regulatory decisions regarding their products. This is articulated in a study published in the journal *Critical Public Health*, which analyzed e-mails between former senior executives at Coca-Cola. Their analysis found that "deliberate" actions were taken by the company to influence scientific evidence and expert opinion, in an effort to push public policy in their favor.

When we see the latest nutrition science story in the news, we need to be skeptical—and look at whether the science is independent or not. If it's not independent, we should look at the source of its funding and consider how this study fits within the larger body of research.

BIG FOOD AND NUTRITION EXPERTS

Many dietitians have partnered up with Big Food, blurring the lines between valid nutritional information and food marketing. Some glaring examples:

The Academy of Nutrition and Dietetics put the first "Kids Eat Right" seal on Kraft Singles (an American cheese snack that isn't more than 51 percent real cheese). Thankfully this was short-lived. Although the Academy and Kraft Foods initially entered into a three-year partnership, they received so much backlash that they were forced to remove the seal from Kraft's processed cheese during the first month.[43]

Frito-Lay once pitched dietitians to advocate Fritos as a good option for a gluten-free diet.[44] Frito-Lay has also sponsored seminars or dietitians in which the company advised dietitians on health trends and nutrition education. Frito-Lay even created an entire website dedicated to nutritionists called SnackSense.com, where they further attempted to convince health professionals that chips are healthy. Here, they told dietitians that "There is no 'junk' in Fritos Original corn chips" and that they fit into a "healthier lifestyle."[45] Registered dietitians are the people who are supposed to be telling us what is healthy to eat—and they are being taught that Fritos are a health food?

Over the years, junk food companies like Nestlé, Hershey's, and PepsiCo have set up exhibit booths at the biggest nutrition conferences in the industry. McDonald's was an official sponsor of the California Academy of Nutrition and Dietetics' annual conferences in 2014 and 2017.[46]

This is ridiculous, right?

When I realized that junk food companies were teaching and catering to health professionals, I was horrified (and some responsible dietitians are horrified as well). However, this isn't a new trend: there's a long list of processed food companies and trade associations that have been accredited to teach continuing education courses to registered dietitians, including General Mills, Kraft, Coca-Cola, and PepsiCo. For instance, Coca-Cola once bragged, "In 2014 alone the number of courses completed by RNs, RDs, pharmacists and other HPs exceeded 300,000, and today more than 40,000 nurses know more about the safety and benefits of low-calorie sweeteners as a direct result of these programs."[47]

And guess what: the industry's plan is working. Some registered dietitians are now touting it's okay to eat Hostess cupcakes if they are in a "100 calorie" pack, drink Crystal Light, or to eat "fresco style" at Taco Bell if you're trying to lose weight.[48]

This would be funny if it wasn't true. And if the lies weren't so dangerous.

HOW THE GOVERNMENT PROMOTES PIZZA HUT

Whether we like it or not, a lot of lobbying goes on in Washington, D.C., and some of the strongest lobbying efforts are made by the food industry. One of the most powerful lobbying groups is the dairy industry, which long ago succeeded in securing dairy as an actual food group in the American diet. In 2006 the dairy lobby triumphed again by not only maintaining dairy as a food group, but in getting a revision in the U.S. Dietary Guidelines to bump up the dairy recommendation from two servings a day to three servings for adults and children. This still stands in the current guidelines, and the exact wording is: "Recommendations are 2 cups (or the equivalent in yogurt or cheese) for children ages 2 to 3 years, 2½ cups for children ages 4 to 8 years, and 3 cups for teens ages 9 to 18 years and for adults."[49]

Tax dollars also help promote unhealthy fast food products like pizza and cheesy sandwiches. Thanks to a government program called "dairy checkoff," the USDA helps market junk food sold by huge restaurant chains as long as it contains dairy products. For instance, the USDA-managed "dairy checkoff" provides funding to Dairy Management Inc., a corporation who collaborates with fast food companies to sell products like a Pizza Hut pan pizza with 25 percent more cheese and McDonald's Egg White Delight McMuffins with 30 percent larger cheese slices. They even once worked with Wendy's to create a Cheddar-Lover's Bacon Cheeseburger that was loaded with two slices of cheddar and draped in cheese sauce. These foods are terrible for us, but the dairy lobby is so powerful that they've persuaded the government that we should be eating more of them.[50]

Let me be clear: I'm not down on dairy. I firmly believe, though, that most Americans should eat less dairy, not more. I also believe that they should be very choosy about where their dairy comes from. The reason? Most dairy foods are laced with hormones, chemicals, and other toxins. On typical farms in the United States, calves are separated from their mothers shortly after birth; this creates a great deal of pain and suffering for the mama cow, causing her to secrete massive amounts of stress hormones that are released into her milk. These toxins are then passed down to us, along with all the other unknown antibiotics, growth hormones, and chemicals the industry uses to produce the milk. I'm pretty sure those fast food chains aren't spending the extra money to ensure their milk comes from the most organic, grass-fed, and humane sources.

Milk is also pasteurized to control bacterial growth. Pasteurization, however, destroys many nutrients found in raw milk. Consider a 2011 study published in *The Journal of Food Protection*, which reported that pasteurization decreases vitamin E and several B vitamins, including B_1, B_2, B_{12}, and folate.[51] The heat also destroys enzymes your body needs for proper digestion. One of these is phosphatase. Without this enzyme, the calcium lingers in your bloodstream and can accumulate in your arteries. As a result, your arteries get stiff and it's more difficult for them to pump blood. Stiff arteries give rise to hypertension (high blood pressure), chest pain, and heart failure.

Lobbying is unbelievably powerful. A startling case occurred not long ago when a government-appointed agency, the American

Egg Board (AEB), tried to crush the vegan food startup Hampton Creek because their blossoming business was a big threat to the multibillion-dollar egg industry.

Representing egg farmers across the U.S., AEB lobbied hard to attack Hampton Creek because it had invented a low-cost, plant-based egg replacement. Hampton Creek is also the maker of Just Mayo, a popular egg-free mayonnaise.

E-mails obtained under the Freedom of Information Act, totaling 600 pages, revealed that the AEB was very worried about Hampton Creek and wanted to drop the hammer on egg-less mayo.[52] In one effort, the AEB tried to get Just Mayo yanked from Whole Foods Market. The U.S. Department of Agriculture's national supervisor of shell eggs suggested that the AEB contact the FDA with their concerns about Just Mayo. The FDA later ruled Just Mayo must change its name. (Whole Foods still sells Just Mayo, and they were able to keep the name Just Mayo.) Furthermore, the e-mails showed they spoke with representatives for Unilever on their false advertising lawsuit against Hampton Creek and had also hired a consultant to examine Hampton Creek's patent for their egg replacer.

Most harrowing of all, the e-mails revealed the presumably joking suggestion that someone contact "some of my old buddies in Brooklyn to pay Mr. Tetrick [Hampton Creek CEO Josh Tetrick] a visit" in response to an e-mail from an AEB member organization executive who asked, "Can we pool our money and put a hit on him?"

And it's not just fights over mayo: there are countless examples of how pressure from Big Food shapes public policy, often with huge consequences. Consider the fight over GMO labeling, which would allow consumers to know which foods contain GMO ingredients. On July 7, 2016, after months of intense lobbying from the farming and processed food industry, the Senate voted 63 to 30 in favor of a sham GMO labeling bill (clearly written to protect Monsanto and the agrochemical and GMO industries) as it allows companies to use QR (quick response) codes to label GMOs in their products, instead of simple words on the package. QR codes are cryptic bar code symbols that require a smartphone equipped with a special app in order to read them, as well as Internet access, as the scanner directs you to a website that provides information about the product. This discriminates against low-income families, minorities, mothers, seniors, the disabled, and those without smartphones. Plus—it's just ludicrous. Wouldn't simple words on the package stating "Contains GMO Ingredients" be easier for everyone?

According to a survey of 800 Americans by the research firm The Mellman Group, only 16 percent of consumers have ever scanned a QR code for any purpose. That's likely because QR code scanning takes time in the store. You have to open the app, scan the product, wait for the web page to load, and select the proper tab for information on GMOs. Who is really going to take the time to do that in the grocery store? On the other hand, it takes seconds to read a text-based label on a package (and we don't need any special equipment). A whopping 88 percent of consumers agree with me and say they'd rather see on-package labeling of GMO foods rather than QR codes. But it doesn't matter what we want—too many of our politicians are more interested in what Monsanto wants.

And it's not just Congress. Many government agencies, including the FDA and the Environmental Protection Agency (EPA), have failed us on so many levels, allowing companies to use and produce dozens of synthetic food additives and agricultural chemicals that are banned or heavily restricted in countries with stronger regulations.

Speaking of the EPA (which is in charge of regulating agricultural chemicals), it was slated to hold four days of public meetings in October 2016 to focus on one key issue: whether or not glyphosate, the world's most widely used herbicide, can cause cancer. Monsanto derives billions in revenue from selling glyphosate, so you probably aren't surprised to hear that they've been telling us it's safe for decades. But these public hearings were going to investigate that claim. Seems like a good idea to me, don't you think? Isn't that why we have the EPA?

But tellingly, the meeting was postponed just four days before it was to begin. Why? Because the agrochemical industry exerted intense pressure. They argued that if the meetings were held, several leading experts should be excluded from participating, to include "any person who has publicly expressed an opinion regarding the carcinogenicity of glyphosate." In other words, the hearings should only proceed if all critical experts were banned from speaking.[53]

As the meetings drew near, CropLife America, a trade group representing Monsanto and other Big Chemical companies, alleged that some panel scientists may be biased against the industry. For example, the group asked that Dr. Kenneth Portier of the American Cancer Society[54] be deeply scrutinized for any "pre-formed conclusions" about glyphosate, and that leading epidemiologist Dr. Peter Infante be completely disqualified from participating at all.[55] This intense lobbying helps explain why the EPA concluded that glyphosate is not carcinogenic,[56] contradicting the findings of the World Health Organization.

To make matters worse, in November 2016, the FDA suspended testing for glyphosate residues in food, breaking an earlier promise.[57] It would have been the FDA's first-ever endeavor to get a handle on just how much of the controversial chemical—deemed a probable carcinogen by the cancer research arm of the World Health Organization[58]—is making its way into our food supply. Shouldn't we know that? Don't we have a *right* to know that? (As we'll learn in Chapter 10, independent labs have conducted their own testing—and the truth about glyphosate in our food is terrifying.)

But maybe I shouldn't have been surprised. As we'll learn in Chapter 3, the FDA has historically been a stumbling block, at least when it comes to getting transparency from the food industry.

GUILTY AS CHARGED!

Everyone shopping for food in a grocery store wants a healthier food system. We all want to buy products that make us feel good, not bad; that help our families flourish; that don't contain ingredients known to cause us harm.

Alas, many of the companies responsible for creating those products on the store shelf have a different goal. They want to make lots of money, which means creating food we can't stop eating even if it's really bad for us. (Bonus points if the processed food is cheap to produce.) The end result is a broken food system, full of unregulated food additives and chemicals that only improve the bottom line of food and biotech companies while damaging our health.

How do these companies get away with it? By telling us lies. By deliberately confusing us, making sure we don't know how to eat right. They will fight anything and everything, from scientific information to independent reports, that threatens their profit margins. They will lobby the government, influence scientists, pay for front groups, and generally do whatever it takes to persuade us to do exactly what independent nutritional science (and even common sense!) tells us *not* to do.

Nutrition really isn't that complicated. We know that we should be eating more whole foods and avoiding junk food and processed foods. Alas, in this world of Big Food propaganda, eating real food that's good for us is bad for business. After all, if we all ate real food . . . Big Food would practically be out of business.

If you find all of this troubling, wait until you learn more about how the food industry, front groups, trade associations, and other guilty parties are *spreading* their lies, inundating us with misinformation and falsehoods about the foods we eat every day.

CHAPTER 2

Spreading Food Lies

For Big Food, it's not enough to invent lies about what we're eating—they need to *spread* those lies, to persuade millions of consumers that highly processed food in boxes, cans, and aluminum foil isn't bad for us.

This chapter is about how they do that. We already know about their huge marketing campaigns, which are designed to trick us into buying their products. (Why else would we spend good money on dyed sugar water with bubbles?) But it turns out Big Food has also invested in more subtle means of spreading their lies, which often involve manipulating the media and paying "experts" to shill for their side.

Look, for instance, at how Coca-Cola uses fitness and nutrition experts to deftly spread a series of dangerous lies about soda, sugar, and calories. According to an expose in the *Dallas Morning News*, Coca-Cola has dozens of dietitians, academics, fitness experts, chefs, and nutritionists on their payroll.[1] When the soda company wants to get out a new message, they lean on these experts to write blogs and articles touting their new drink. That's exactly what happened after Coca-Cola introduced smaller soda cans. At the behest of the company, dietitians and nutritionists wrote numerous pieces (several of which ended up in major newspapers) that celebrated the smaller cola cans as a healthy treat. Even worse, the articles never disclosed that they were essentially paid advertisements.[2]

Are you kidding me? This is blatant misinformation—soda is *never* a healthy treat, not even in a smaller serving size—and it's gross that the so-called experts never disclose why they're suddenly so supportive of Coca-Cola products.

In many instances, Coca-Cola was the main sponsor of science journalism conferences, allowing the company to plant story ideas that later appeared on CNN and in major newspapers. Coca-Cola's sponsorship was hidden from journalists. According to the *BMJ*, these journalism conferences delivered far more B.S. for the buck than conventional advertisements.[3] Why? Because they delivered lies that felt true. And they were *everywhere*.

I have to admit that, for me, the spreading of Big Food lies is a personal issue. That's because I've been a frequent target of corporate attacks, as their shills try to discredit me and the Food Babe Army. While the criticisms can sting, I also know that they are a testament to our success. The more powerful we get, and the more companies we convince to remove additives and chemicals, the more Big Food tries to stop us. But they can't.

My first memorable experience with their attacks occurred, not surprisingly, right after a big win for the Food Babe Army. We'd just forced Subway to remove the controversial chemical azodicarbonamide (the yoga mat chemical) from its bread. We had also succeeded in getting the largest beer company in the world—Anheuser-Busch—to publish the ingredients in their beer for the first time in history. Our work was making front page news all over the world.

When you put yourself out there, you have to be ready to deal with the negatives as well as the positives—and with the haters along with the supporters. And I've got thick skin. But I wasn't prepared for the coordinated attacks that took advantage of the biased media. Big Food hasn't just mastered the art of deception and distraction using lobbyists, front groups, paid scientists, and other experts; they're also really good at manipulating the media to deliver messages that support food industry positions and refute information that might challenge their status quo.

The ugly truth is that many media outlets have become nothing more than a spin factory for Big Food.

CONTROVERSY OVER COCONUT OIL

Not long ago, the headlines blared:

- "Coconut oil isn't healthy. It's never been healthy."—*USA Today*[4]

- "Nutrition experts warn coconut oil is on par with beef fat, butter."—*Chicago Tribune*[5]

- "This popular health food is worse for you than pork lard."—*Daily Star*[6]

- "Coconut oil isn't as healthy as we thought, according to depressing new study."—*Elite Daily*[7]

If you read these headlines, you probably wondered, as I did: "What the heck is going on? I thought coconut oil was healthy."

For the record, I still am convinced that coconut oil is healthy. I use it to bake cookies and to "butter" my popcorn. It's a regular part of my diet, and I consider it to be one of the best oils to eat—period. If you dig into the *unbiased* scientific literature, you'll find out a lot about its therapeutic benefits: protection against heart disease, cancer, obesity, diabetes, and various degenerative illnesses.

So why coconut oil's sudden fall from grace?

That's what I wanted to know too.

PRESCRIPTION FOR COLLUSION

A little digging on my part unearthed the source: the American Heart Association (AHA). In 2017, it released a jaw-dropping "Presidential Advisory," in which a writing panel composed of experts recommended that we avoid coconut oil, stating that it is high in saturated fat and raises "bad" cholesterol levels—which the AHA believes leads to heart disease (although there is credible evidence to the contrary).[8] The advisory went on to recommend that we swap coconut oil with olive oil or . . . corn oil.

Oh, no! Corn oil is exactly the oil we should be avoiding, along with soybean and canola oils. I've heavily researched these oils. As I noted in Chapter 1, they go through an insane amount of processing with chemical solvents, steamers, neutralizers, de-waxers, bleach, and deodorizers before they end up in the bottle. These cooking oils are also very high in omega-6 fatty acids, which are known to promote inflammation in the body. Chronic inflammation is a real killer, increasing the risk of heart disease, type 2 diabetes, and Alzheimer's disease.[9] These oils are also strongly linked to cancer and are typically derived from genetically modified crops contaminated with Roundup herbicide, made by Monsanto.

But don't take my word for it. In 2017, a large statistical study in *Nutrition Journal* revealed that replacing saturated fats with polyunsaturated fats (like corn oil) is not likely to reduce risk of heart disease one bit, nor influence cholesterol levels.[10] If you look at the countries that consume the most coconut oil, they've also got some of the lowest rates of heart disease . . . what does that tell you?

The AHA is a nonprofit organization with a mission to "build healthier lives free of cardiovascular disease and stroke." But I join many other critics in believing that the AHA is not true to this calling. For example, that Presidential Advisory has since been widely criticized for using "cherry-picked" studies—and rightly so. The AHA's main conclusions were based on only four trials, with the latest one done in 1971, making them "ancient" by the standards of modern scientific research.[11]

The AHA Presidential Advisory writing panel was also blasted because it included a member whose previous research was funded by numerous drug companies, many of whom make cholesterol pills: Amarin, Amgen, AstraZeneca (maker of the statin Crestor), Eli Lilly, GlaxoSmithKline, Merck, Pfizer,

Regeneron/Sanofi, and Takeda.[12] Another member was previously funded by the Ag Canada and Canola Oil Council,[13] while another had previously received consulting fees from several drug companies including Abbott, Amgen, Eli Lilly, and Merck. Another researcher has received significant research support from Unilever (maker of Hellmann's mayonnaise made with soybean oil).[14]

All of this adds up to major conflicts of interest, with the food industry in bed with a medical organization, operating under the guise of truth and objectivity.

Lucky Charms Are Good for the Heart (and Other Advertising Sins)

Big Food will heavily advertise its products; that's a given. But let me tell you about another sneaky tactic: medical endorsements from health organizations. They know we trust these organizations, which is precisely why they're so determined to use them to help spread their lies.

The American Heart Association is a perfect example of how this works. The AHA has a program in which it allows a "heart check" seal to be put on approved foods that are low in saturated fat and cholesterol. Those foods are considered certified by the AHA. Although a lot of healthy foods are certified (avocados and fresh sweet potatoes, to name two), there are many foods on the list that are loaded with sugar and other nasty ingredients:[15]

- Pepperidge Farm Whole Grain Honey Wheat Bread with added sugar, soybean oil, and two additives that contain trans fats (DATEM and monoglycerides).

- Frescados Tomato Basil Wrap made with hydrogenated cottonseed oil, artificial food dyes, and cellulose gum.

- Westsoy Organic Original SoyMilk sweetened with brown rice syrup, containing a whopping 12 grams of sugar per serving (the unsweetened version is certified too, but it only has 3 grams sugar).

- Minute Maid Frozen Concentrate Orange Juice that has the same amount of sugar as a Coke.

- Classic Creations Flake Style Imitation Crab Meat made with artificial sugars, artificial flavors, and carrageenan.

Although they don't anymore, the AHA once certified fat-free chocolate milk and Cocoa Puffs, Lucky Charms, and Trix cereals. (Who knew eating artificially colored and sugar-filled marshmallows for breakfast was good for your heart?) They also certify heavily processed deli meats full of sugar, salt, and preservatives, like heavily processed Boar's Head products.[16] Both of these categories of food (sugary foods and processed deli meats) are associated with a dramatically increased risk of heart disease, according to research from Harvard.[17]

In one of these studies, scientists said this: "Over the course of the 15-year study on added sugar and heart disease, participants who took in 25 percent or more of their daily calories as sugar were more than twice as likely to die from heart disease as those whose diets included less than 10 percent added sugar."[18]

And researchers from the Harvard T. H. Chan School of Public Health found that eating processed meat, such as bacon, sausage, or processed deli meats, was associated with a 42 percent higher risk of heart disease.[19]

Why, then, is the AHA certifying sugary foods and processed deli meats that are quite clearly bad for the heart? Maybe because there's a financial hitch to this: Companies making these products and dozens more insanely processed foods have each paid thousands of dollars in fees to use the AHA's seal. They're willing to pay for the obvious reason: according to the AHA's own market research, the heart-check symbol helps sell food.

Please recognize squarely where the AHA's loyalty lies; don't just toss certain foods in your cart because they display a heart-check seal. Looking at where the AHA's revenue comes from, you've got to question the veracity of their opinions on what constitutes "heart healthy" food.

I for one do not trust the AHA—can you tell? Last year, I was invited to join some celebrities, including a few of my favorite NFL players, at a fundraiser, an even that I would have loved to go to. I declined the invitation because the event was sponsored by the AHA. It killed me to decline the opportunity, but it was the right thing to do.

I know it's frustrating when there is so much conflicting health information being fired at us from all directions. How can we know what to believe? How can we know we're getting accurate advice? Who should we listen to? How can we expect to get healthy?

When it comes to health information, we must always consider the source (and examine it well!). Even if advice seems to come from perfectly respectable organizations on the surface, like the American Heart Association, research who they are, who funds their work, and what types of health claims they've made in the past. This is something I do when reading health-related articles. In today's age of political and industry propaganda, it is imperative that you take this step and thus become your own health advocate.

Those coconut oil headlines are just a single example of how Big Food can twist and distort the truth about food. It's time to sort through the constant stream of misinformation, mixed messages, and claims that stretch, bend, or simply invent the truth in the media.

SLANTED NEWS

Soon after I exposed the ingredients in Starbucks most infamous drink—the Pumpkin Spice Latte—there was a media firestorm. My blog post made headlines from *USA Today*[20] to Fox News.[21] My phone was ringing off the hook while my blog post on the subject went viral on social media, with more than a million shares. The major press up until this point had been generally positive about our work—this was when everything began to change.

Harsh critics suddenly materialized out of nowhere. It was like nothing I had seen before. They started trolling my Facebook posts and angrily tweeting at me; I received hateful e-mails and letters. Every single day.

But the most troubling criticisms started to appear in major media articles, as journalists began quoting "experts" without disclosing their conflicts of interest and ties to the industry. Consider an article that appeared on *The Salt*, an NPR blog.[22] The journalist, Maria Godoy, reached out to me in this e-mail:

> Hi, Vani, I want to speak with you about growing criticism among scientists of the claims you make about food additives. As you know, you've been accused of distorting the science in some cases, and as your profile grows, it's likely that so, too, will these criticisms. I want to hear your response to these criticisms. Would you be available for a telephone interview? This would be for a story for The Salt, NPR's food vertical. Thanks in advance for your time. Regards, Maria Godoy, NPR

Naturally, I wanted to do the interview. I wanted to clear up any confusion and give my perspective, especially since I am very meticulous about the research I rely on. In my writing, I use a variety of published scientific papers, interviews with experts, studies, and opinions from noteworthy and respected public interest groups. We are still learning the impact of the food we eat—much of it hasn't even been studied—and thousands of chemicals in our food supply remain untested. So much new information is being discovered every single day. And that information is constantly changing, increasing the uncertainty of concerned consumers. So of course I wanted to do this interview.

But my then publisher said no. Their rationale? They wanted me to wait to do interviews until my first book (*The Food Babe Way*) was published.

I later found this to be a huge mistake. I got blindsided.

Not only did Godoy move forward with the piece, but she wrote a completely biased, negative view about the campaigns and research I had presented in my writings. The title of the article was "Is the Food Babe a Fearmonger? Scientists Are Speaking

Out." Guess what: only one critic interviewed was actually a food scientist.

After Godoy's article came out, I was shocked by the people she interviewed. Here are two examples of the figures she relied on:

Kavin Senapathy. Neither a scientist nor a doctor, Senapathy calls herself a "science defender" on social media. She cofounded the organization March Against Myths About Modification (MAMyths), which is a "partner" of Biology Fortified, a website that advocates strongly for GMOs, and has on at least one occasion worked with the PR group Cornell Alliance for Science.[23] She attends marches wearing an "I Love GMOs" t-shirt and protests talks given by anti-GMO food activists. She had written for several pro-GMO blogs. She has been photographed with Monsanto representatives and their PR firm reps. She once e-mailed me for comment on a story she was writing but refused to answer my questions about her conflicts of interest.

Senapathy has taken a big interest in me personally. She spends a significant amount of time criticizing me and the work of the Food Babe Army. She acted as the spokesperson for a Facebook page that was created solely to criticize and parody me all day long, every day, sometimes in extremely offensive ways. She even cowrote an entire book about me called *The Fear Babe*. You've got to wonder why she spends so much of her time focused on discrediting me.

In more recent years, Senapathy has published several articles in *Forbes* and on its website, which reaches millions. In it, she spews hate for organic food and farming, and bashes non-GMO food activists like me repeatedly with articles such as:

"3 Tactics Donald Trump Shares with Dr. Oz, The Food Babe, and Other Snake Oil Salesmen"—*Forbes*, 10/5/16.[24]

"The Food Babe Is a Bully and Cotton Incorporated Isn't Going To Take It"—*Forbes*, 5/27/2016.[25]

"Del Monte Joins Food Babe Army, Shuns Fruit-Saving Technology"—*Forbes*, 4/5/2016.[26]

"The Toxic 'Chemical Hypocrisy' Of Food Babe, Joseph Mercola and Mark Hyman"—*Forbes*, 12/3/2015.[27]

In Senapathy's controversial articles, her sources are PR operatives and people who are paid to protect the profits of Big Food and GMO companies. For instance, she cites:

- U.S. Farmers and Ranchers Alliance (funded by DuPont and Monsanto[28] and run by the PR firm Ketchum)

- Cotton Incorporated (a trade group for cotton growers who have received technology from Monsanto)[29]

- An advisor for the Calorie Control Council (a trade group for artificial sweetener manufacturers)

Are these groups "independent experts"? Absolutely not.

Senapathy got her start at *Forbes* co-writing several pieces with Henry Miller, a former FDA employee who is associated with several front groups that ferociously defend the use of GMOs and pesticides. His résumé includes accolades from Philip Morris for defending the tobacco industry. Miller had been writing pro-GMO articles for *Forbes* for more than 10 years; however, in August 2017 his association with *Forbes* abruptly ended. The reason? A *New York Times* investigation uncovered that Monsanto ghostwrote Miller's article defending its glyphosate-containing herbicide Roundup.[30] Nowhere in the *Forbes* article did Miller disclose his relationship with Monsanto, nor the fact that the company wrote the piece for him. After this came to light, *Forbes* took action. While *Forbes* yanked the article from its website (along with other pieces he coauthored with Senapathy), you've got to wonder how many people it misled in the years it was online. Monsanto later admitted that their "scientists have on occasion collaborated with Dr. Miller on other pieces," so this article was apparently not an isolated incident.[31]

Dr. Kevin Folta. You may recall Folta from the previous chapter, as one of the experts quoted in a *New York Times* hit piece about me who was later outed in the same publication for having ties to Monsanto. This university professor in horticultural sciences has for years claimed to be "an independent scientist" with "no financial ties to any of the BigAg companies that make transgenic crops," yet according to his own website, TalkingBiotech.com, he has received support for his outreach efforts from several pro-GMO and biotech industry groups. His industry sponsors have included:[32]

- Croplife Canada—a large trade group that includes Monsanto, Bayer, DuPont, and a who's who list of biotech and chemical corporations[33]

- The American Seed Trade Association—self-described "advocates for the industry" led by corporate executives from agricultural giants like Bayer[34]

- The Oregon Farm Bureau—a powerful lobbying group for the industry and Big Ag[35]

- Manitoba Canola Growers—funded by the canola check-off program; canola oil is a major GMO crop[36]

- The Florida Fertilizer and Agrichemical Association —an industry trade group for makers of pesticides and herbicides; Folta received a $5,000 honorarium from them in 2016[37]

- Farm & Food Care Saskatchewan—sponsored by GMO and synthetic agrichemical companies DEKALB (a Monsanto brand), Croplife Canada (trade group), and Cargill[38]

- Great Lakes Crop Summit—an event sponsored by Bayer, DuPont, DEKALB, and BASF[39]

- The Institute of Food Technologists—an organization that represents food scientists who produced the GMO industry propaganda film *Food Evolution*

Considering this list, it's hard to believe that Dr. Kevin Folta is truly independent and isn't swayed by these industry sponsors. Even more so in 2017, Folta openly disclosed research funding from Bayer AG (who recently acquired Monsanto). A funding letter obtained by U.S. Right to Know shows that Bayer sent Folta a grant for 50,000 euros (about $58,000 in U.S. dollars).[40]

Folta has taken the opportunity to jab me at every turn. Check out the following e-mail thread between him and the NPR reporter, which I obtained via the Freedom of Information Act:[41]

Maria Godoy: "I'm interested in writing a post for our food blog, *The Salt* (a product of the science desk) about the science community's backlash against the "Food Babe." I came across your blog posts from last week about Vani Hari's appearance at the University of Florida and was hoping to speak with you about the event."

Folta: "I would love to discuss it. My blood pressure is just getting back to the range where I can safely lift heavy objects."

This exchange occurred on October 28, 2014, prior to the publication of Godoy's article on December 4, 2014.

Look, I'm all in favor of honest debate. Given all the uncertainty and contradictory evidence, I think reasonable people can disagree about food and nutrition issues. When I make a mistake, I try to correct it.

However, I don't think it's helpful when people with clear conflicts of interest fail to disclose them. We have a right to know who takes money from Big Food and Big Ag, because that can help us evaluate their evidence and arguments. (As we saw in the last chapter, research groups funded by the food industry are far more likely to publish results that support their marketing goals.) And when journalists publish one-sided hit pieces, and never highlight the biases of their sources, they are playing right into the industry's hands.

JOURNALISTS FOR HIRE

At this point, I'm pretty cynical about the relationship between Big Food and the media. I know that money talks, and that Big Food has a lot of it. But even I'm still amazed at the sheer brazenness with which commercial interests try to influence journalists.

In 2016, Monsanto picked up the tab—including airfare, hotels, meals, tote bags, notebooks, and pencils—to bring 20 journalists to the company's St. Louis headquarters.[42] The purpose of the four-day trip was to counter public perceptions that Monsanto is involved only in GMOs, and that it doesn't care about food safety and the environment. The goal of the junket, of course, was to generate positive news stories about the company. As I've noted, Monsanto is the leading producer, worldwide, of GMOs, and maker of the controversial weed killer Roundup. It needs all the good press it can get.

Corporate-sponsored junkets like this are nothing new. They came into existence in the 1930s when film studios invited reporters to movie screenings and parties with actors and actresses. Since then, junkets have become a mainstay of many industries. Increasingly, however, they are being used to corrupt our food news.

But junkets are only one of the ways money shapes your news. Big Food is also notorious for paying dietitians and other experts to write positively about food products—and bash competing interests. You see this all the time in the David and Goliath–type battle between organic food producers and conventional growers.

DIRTY DOZEN UNDER ATTACK

One of the most egregious pieces of anti-organic reporting appeared in the *Washington Post* under the headline "A diet rich in fruits and vegetables outweighs the risks of pesticides."[43] The article was written by Cara Rosenbloom, a registered dietitian. Rosenbloom is also the founder of Words to Eat By, a full-service nutrition communications company, in which she writes articles for magazines, blogs, newspapers and websites. She also engages in "Strategy and brainstorming sessions with PR and marketing agencies to facilitate content development, media campaigns and new product launches."[44]

Her article in the *Washington Post* claimed that the Dirty Dozen and the Clean Fifteen—lists researched by the Environmental Working Group (EWG) that rank fruits and vegetables by their pesticide residue loads—are "being questioned for their scientific validity—may be doing more harm than good."[45] The article steers the reader away from organic food as the best choice and states: "Misinformation about pesticides breeds fear and confusion, and many find it easier to skip fresh produce altogether." The messaging in the article is to forget pesticides and eat fruits and vegetables, regardless of whether they're organic or not. Her list of writing samples shows she writes regularly for *Washington Post*, one of the most widely read publications in the U.S.

Notably, Rosenbloom's article was promptly shared by the Big Ag industry front group Alliance for Food and Farming in their e-mail newsletter, stating, "Today the *Washington Post* ran an article titled 'A Diet Rich in Fruits and Vegetables Outweighs the Risks of Pesticides.' The story reflected Alliance for Food and Farming messaging and included content from our website safefruitsandveggies.com and recent press release."

Although this article appeared in a major media outlet, it included no rebuttal or comment from the EWG on their Dirty Dozen list. If they'd been asked, I imagine the EWG would have told them how they rigorously analyzed tests performed by the USDA that revealed "that nearly 70 percent of samples of 48 types of conventional produce were contaminated with residues of one or more pesticides. USDA researchers found a total of 178 different pesticides and pesticide breakdown products on the thousands of produce samples they analyzed. The pesticide residues remained on fruits and vegetables even after they were washed and, in some cases, peeled."[46] How is this invalid science or "misinformation"? Inconvenient facts are still facts.

EWG is a nonprofit, nonpartisan organization dedicated to protecting human health and the environment. (See the latest version of the EWG's Dirty Dozen and Clean 15 on page 195.) It has its own team of scientists, policy experts, and others who do exhaustive research to make sure someone is standing up for public health when government and industry won't.

Of course, that used to be the job of the news media. But as we've seen, that's no longer the case.

A TANGLED WEB: DESIGNED TO DECEIVE

You have surely encountered this phenomenon online, but may not have recognized it as an industry tactic because it is so stealthy. In what has been called "astroturfing,"[47] the industry hires groups of people to leave comments online in an effort to appear as though they are part of a large grassroots movement that stands firmly on one side of an issue. (Just as astroturf is fake grass that's supposed to look natural, astroturfing involves fake comments that imitate the look and feel of real grassroots supporters.) As can be expected, I have been the target of several astroturfing campaigns, often appearing in the comment sections of Facebook after I launch a successful campaign. After you've seen it a few times, it becomes glaringly obvious what is happening. Let me give you an example from one of the first big astroturfing campaigns directed toward me (which ultimately helped bring light to the phenomenon).

When *Experience Life* magazine asked me to be on the cover, I was pretty excited, as it's one of the few health magazines I read on a regular basis. And I had so much fun doing the shoot and interview—I felt like a movie star for the day, with my clothes set out for me and my hair and makeup done by famous makeup artists who had worked with some of the top actresses in Hollywood. (The photographer had just photographed Michelle Obama the week before.) What made the experience even cooler is that I wasn't a celebrity. I was an activist.

When the issue hit the stores, I took a trip to Barnes and Noble to see it. At first, I was on cloud nine. But my excitement soon turned into horror. I discovered that an astroturfing campaign had begun, as comment sections on *Experience Life*'s Facebook page suddenly filled up with hundreds of negative comments about my cover. These astroturfers also went to *Experience Life*'s Amazon page and wrote 136 one-star reviews, driving their ranking down from 4½ stars to 2½ stars in a matter of days. This was so egregious because *Experience Life* depends upon their ratings for sales. I was incredibly sad that this was happening to a great magazine just because I was on the cover, exposing the truth about the food industry. The purpose of this astroturfing campaign, of course, was to make sure that no other magazines would ever have me on the cover again (they'd see that if they put me on the cover, they'd be punished). This is how they stifle our message.

At the time, I wanted to hide under a rock. This magazine had taken a courageous stand by putting me on the cover, and now it was being attacked. Fortunately, *Experience Life* noticed what was happening and made a very bold statement on their Facebook page about astroturfing: "Over the weekend, we received an unusually large influx of negative Facebook comments regarding our October cover subject, Vani Hari (a.k.a. The Food Babe). As a whole, these comments bear the earmarks of an industry-coordinated response—one designed to appear as though it is coming from individual consumers, but that is motivated and subsidized by a behind-the-scenes special interest."[48]

This only further angered the astroturfers, but I'm glad *Experience Life* understood what was happening and ultimately ended up covering the topic of astroturfing in a piece called "Turf Wars":

> These campaigns are designed to make it appear that an issue has widespread public support (or public opposition) even if it doesn't. If a campaign sows enough doubt, excitement, or skepticism about a contentious

issue or individual, it can shape the opinions of real people. And that's the primary goal.[49]

Knowing that this can happen has made me extremely wary of comment sections on social media, blog posts, and even news sites. When you see dozens or hundreds of comments that make similar statements, go on the attack, and all appear at once (like a mob), there's a good chance you're looking at an example of astroturfing.

We know, for instance, plaintiff's attorneys claim in court documents that Monsanto has a program called "Let Nothing Go," which is designed to leave no critical comment about them unanswered. As was noted in a court document, Monsanto, "through a series of third parties, employs individuals who appear to have no connection to the industry, who in turn post positive comments on news articles and Facebook posts, defending Monsanto, its chemicals, and GMOs."[50] That's textbook astroturfing.

I believe that having food that's safe and free of additives is not very controversial—the vast majority of Americans want exactly that. But if you read the comments on *Experience Life*, or on nearly any article that criticizes Big Food, you'd probably think that most Americans want soda full of sugar and chemicals, unlabeled genetically modified ingredients, and lots of additives. Don't let them fool you.

What to Do When You Witness an Astroturfing Campaign

Remember: astroturfing is used to create shame in sharing content online (so we will stop) and to create the illusion that there are negativity and ignorance around the good-food movement. They want to create confusion so you never know who to trust or what to believe. Here's what to do next time you witness it online:

- Call it out for what it is. Use this as an opportunity to educate others about astroturfing. Making people aware of this tactic takes away its effectiveness.

- Share a positive result to counter negative comments. For example, you could say how awesome you feel giving up processed foods and how paying attention to what's in your food has helped you and your family.

- There is no reason to engage with astroturfers online. You can block or ban them from your social media accounts if necessary. Bless them and move on.

SILENCING ACTIVISTS TO STIFLE THE TRUTH

Sometimes, instead of spreading lies, those working to keep the status quo will do everything in their power to prevent activists from getting out the truth about what is really in our food. This has happened to me and countless other activists in the food movement. It has even happened to respected scientists who are breaking rank and speaking out about the industry. This is not a new tactic; Rachel Carson, a pioneering and outspoken activist in the 1960s, was prominently attacked in this way as well. One of the main ways they silence activists is by using astroturfing (and sometimes threats) to prevent us from speaking at events. I was once the victim of this while preparing to give a talk in the beautiful state of Hawaii.

Hawaii is a hotbed of research and development of chemically intensive genetically modified crops and a testing ground for many experimental chemicals; it is essentially "ground zero" for agrichemical companies. I was invited to come speak there by the Hawaii Center for Food Safety (Hawaii CFS) for an event called "The Ethics of Eating." This is the Hawaii chapter of the Center for Food Safety (CFS), a nonprofit organization that promotes organic and sustainable agriculture. They fight back against the corrupt food system with petitions and have bravely taken legal action to force our government to create stronger regulations in regard to GMOs and chemicals that are harming our bodies, the environment, and farm animals. Much of the work Hawaii CFS is doing is focused on the public health impacts of the pesticides and herbicides used on GMOs, and because of this, they are heavily targeted by the biotech companies who are profiting off of these chemicals and technologies. The people who work with CFS are very well respected and fearless activists in an increasingly aggressive climate.

I was thrilled that CFS invited me to come speak at the event, yet I had no idea what absolute chaos would soon ensue. As soon as my upcoming appearance was announced, the Big Ag industry quickly engaged and astroturfing began on the Hawaii CFS Facebook page. CFS suddenly began receiving hundreds of insulting and inflammatory comments, mainly criticizing me personally, characterizing me as "hilariously uninformed" and "a crazy food blogger," and accusing Hawaii CFS of promoting "pseudoscience" and "fearmongering" for bringing me in to speak. The astroturfing was unprecedented. As the director of Hawaii CFS, Ashley Lukens, Ph.D., put it, "Vani's visit to Hawai'i would unleash the most powerful display of the pro-GMO public relations machine that I have witnessed since taking my position with CFS."[51]

This just goes to show the great lengths the industry will go to in an attempt to silence activists and make it difficult for anyone to ever ask me to speak again. They were defaming me in an attempt to harm my future speaking engagements—but they didn't stop there.

Approximately 24 hours before I was scheduled to take the stage, I was informed by Hawaii CFS that a pro-GMO and satire activist group I mentioned earlier, March Against Myths About Modification (MAMyths), had launched an aggressive campaign to sabotage the event.

Although the tickets to the event were free, there were a limited number available, as the venue could only accommodate a certain number of people. When word spread that I was coming to speak, MAMyths asked their followers to reserve blocks of tickets using fake names and fake e-mails so the event would appear to be sold out and I would be speaking to an empty venue. On their Facebook page they announced, "Join us in reserving seats! Free tickets available RIGHT NOW and you can get up to 4 of these limited seats for your friends. Who doesn't want to see the Food Babe speak in person?! #noShow Protips: Order on a future date other than today. Use a disposable email address like mailinator.com (check the alternative domains on front page)." They also suggested using a "random name generator" to get through any controls on tickets.

Their followers proceeded to reserve over 1,500 tickets using names like "Fraud Babe," "Organic is Dumb," "Susi Cream-cheese," and "Harriett Tubman" from proxied IP addresses outside of Hawaii and overseas in the United Kingdom, Australia, China, Thailand, Germany, Sweden, and the Netherlands. They were ultimately unsuccessful because Hawaii CFS discovered where these bogus requests were coming from and was able to easily cancel their tickets. Although MAMyths was trying to destroy the event in a very offensive manner, thankfully the CFS event in Hawaii turned out to be a huge success (granted, CFS had to hire extra security). We had a packed house, with some in standing room only!

BEWARE WHERE THE INTERNET LEADS YOU

Food companies increasingly utilize the Internet and social media to generate brand buzz and boost sales. More than ever before, we learn to cook, save recipes, plan our meals, purchase food, and share food tips with others via websites, Facebook, apps, or blogs.

But you should be wary. Many websites look legitimate but are really digital fronts for Big Food. GMOAnswers.com, for instance, is a joint initiative by the very companies who make GMO seeds and pesticides. While the website asserts that it is committed to transparency about the use of GMOs in agriculture, it's really a vehicle to promote GMOs and pesticides, run by the PR firm Ketchum and funded by the GMO companies.[52] It is not credible at all.

And then there are the many food company–sponsored websites geared to lure kids into the world of junk food. They can log on to Cheetos.com, for example, and watch the brand's mascot, Chester Cheetah, in all sorts of entertaining videos, or play games to earn prizes.

In fact, many of the top food brands that target children through TV ads also have websites geared toward kids and teens. This is scary stuff, especially when you consider that around 9 million young people between the ages of 6 and 19 are overweight and at a greater risk of heart disease and diabetes. It took decades of hard work before the tobacco industry was forced to stop marketing to kids. My hope is that one day, we might also regulate the ability of soda and junk food companies to target our youngest eaters.

I think we can all agree that no one should grow up on a diet of soda and Cheetos.

NATIVE ADVERTISING: HIDDEN IN PLAIN SIGHT

You've seen this tactic daily, but probably don't even realize it. That's by design: native advertising is when ads are interwoven with web content to match the look and feel of a particular website. In short, it's a means of disguising the ad, making it seem less like a paid commercial and more like all the other content on the site. On television, this type of advertising takes on the form of an "infomercial," while in print media it is called an "advertorial."

To understand the impact of these native ads, look at WebMD,[53] the most visited health site on the web. A recent sponsored video on the site by Walgreens encouraged people to continue taking their prescription heart medications—and to make sure to visit their local Walgreens, of course. Another video sponsored by Humira (a prescription medicine for psoriasis) was essentially an advertisement for the drug featuring a dermatologist. In the past, Monsanto was a buyer of native ads on WebMD and had crafted a number of sponsored ads that looked like real content rather than marketing, using WebMD's influence to serve its own agenda.[54]

Knowing that WebMD is considered a trusted source for health information on the Internet, Monsanto has attempted to enlist academics to write articles for WebMD so that "search algorithms" would pick up their content when searched by consumers online. For example, private e-mails obtained via a USRTK FOIA request show that in 2015 Monsanto pitched University of Florida scientist Kevin Folta to submit a blog post to WebMD on the safety of GMO technology. In the e-mail written by Monsanto's Lisa Drake, Dr. Folta was asked to "Please consider insert [sic] the word 'labeling' somewhere in the content in order to get search algorithms to pick it up." (Folta has since claimed he never wrote the piece.)[55]

During this period of time in 2015, GMO labeling was a hot button issue, which Monsanto was trying to stop regulatory action on. Enlisting an "independent" scientist to write an article for WebMD could have bolstered their efforts at stopping GMO labeling.

This is a good reminder to examine carefully who is writing or sponsoring the content you find online—even on the most widely used websites in the world.

PAID ADVOCACY: WIKIPEDIA

Right before my first book was published, someone created a Wikipedia page about me. At first, the page seemed benign and I paid little attention to it. Eventually, though, my page was hijacked by a group of editors who manipulated the content dramatically. Suddenly, my Wikipedia profile made me sound like a crazy person. It stated I was a conspiracy theorist and a hypocrite selling the poisons that I was lobbying against. (A complete lie.) Several editors tried removing positive attributes about me, such as being a *New York Times* best-selling author and a successful consumer advocate. They rewrote my profile, emphasizing criticisms and citing critics known to be pro-GMO and pro-corporation—while removing any mention of all the doctors, nutritionists, and other noted experts who support my work and my cause.

This group of editors watched my page like a hawk—and still does. I've been told that if anyone goes there and tries to make an edit that puts me in a positive light it is swiftly removed, often within minutes. It's pretty crazy.

I watched my Wikipedia page get overrun and realized there was little I could do. You see, per Wikipedia guidelines in general, you are not permitted to edit a page about yourself. Of course, I wondered where these editors that had taken over my page came from. And why were they spending so much time guarding the content? Was someone paying them to do this? That seemed like a logical explanation.

A few months later at a book signing in northern California, a gentleman approached me and confessed that he was one of those Wikipedia editors. He told me he had been hired by a PR firm to make sure my entry would be cast in a negative light. He apologized profusely to me after learning my story and using some of my advice to regain his health. I was stunned. Up to that point, I had no idea that Wikipedia is frequently manipulated by the corporate world.

An investigation by *The Atlantic* confirmed that many people, groups, and corporations resort to paying freelancers, PR firms, and other Wiki "experts" to make edits to the site. *The Atlantic* article stated: ". . . the site has enormous reach, and the information it contains makes its way to nearly everyone, from consumers to policymakers to people Googling innocuous questions on their phones. Even minor changes in wording have the potential to influence public perception and, naturally, how millions of dollars are spent. What this means for marketers is that Wikipedia is yet another place to establish an online presence."[56]

A search on Upwork (a freelance job posting site) turns up several Wikipedia editors for hire, asking upward of $50 per hour. Not a bad gig, huh? While Wikipedia has rules put in place that are supposed to discourage paid editing, *The Atlantic* reported:

> Many people who work within companies' public relations departments are inexperienced in the ways of Wikipedia, and some firms look outside of their ranks for

editing help . . . 'Wikipedia writing is like no other writing,' says Mike Wood, a freelancer who makes a living editing Wikipedia pages for clients, referring to the site's tireless pursuit of a neutral tone. Wood has set up his own website, and scores of other Wikipedia editors for hire await on freelance websites such as Elance. He says he works with highly visible people and companies, who pay him anywhere from $400 to $1,000 per article, but he won't name names, for fear that someone might seek out and dismantle the Wikipedia pages of his clients.[57]

What this means for companies, including Big Food, is that Wikipedia is yet another place to sway consumers and spread lies. How, then, can we separate truth from fiction?

I suggest that you use Wikipedia as a starting place, not as the ultimate word. Keep in mind that human beings with biases (and in some cases, paid agendas) have posted the information you are reading.

Then dig deeper into other sources of research. The footnotes and references given in Wikipedia can help you. Read the listed academic papers and review articles, and then look for the disclosure statement of the scientists and authors; find websites and blogs that deliver complex and comprehensive insights into your topic.

The moral of the story: Wikipedia readers, beware.

SNIFF OUT THE TRUTH

As you can see, information released to the public is often corrupted by commercial interests. As I've hopefully made clear, we must stay skeptical and think critically. We shouldn't believe everything we read.

To separate the truth from the bull, I have the following suggestions.

- Scrutinize the source of the information, the source's possible agenda, and the evidence provided in the message. If possible, ask: Is the evidence science-based? Who funded the science? Does the evidence logically support the claims being made? Does it seem like relevant facts or context have been left out? Remember that commercial pressures shape the form and content of research and news—and exert massive influence.

- Determine whether all representative viewpoints, for and against an issue, are presented. If everything is squarely on one side of an issue, you can bet that you are not getting the whole story.

- Diversify your sources of news and information.

- Check to see if the headline matches the facts in the story. If not, it could be a biased, less-than-truthful story.

- Determine whether the story can also be found on several credible news outlets. (Try Internet searching the story headline or people's names associated with the article to see if there are other news outlets running the story or refuting the claims.)

Someone once said "A lie can travel halfway around the world while the truth is putting on its shoes."

It's often hard to figure out the facts. However, when it comes to your diet and health, I think it's absolutely worth investing the extra effort and time to determine what's real and what's not. At the end of the day, it's nobody else's responsibility to tell you what's true. You alone are responsible for the news you consume. If you want to be healthy—and don't we all?—determining which foods are actually good for you is imperative.

On that subject: in the next part of this book, we'll look at the specific food lies we're being fed—and how to avoid their consequences. Before we can learn the truth about healthy food, we have to learn to avoid those foods that are making us sick.

Because they're everywhere.

Part II

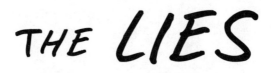

THE LIES

CHAPTER 3

Us versus the Rest of the World

If you really want to understand how broken the American food system is, you just need to walk into a grocery store in Europe and look at the ingredients in their products. Pick up a bottle of Mountain Dew in the U.K., for instance. You'll find that it gets its bright yellow color simply from beta carotene (a natural color derived from carrots and other plants). Meanwhile, PepsiCo sells a very different version of Mountain Dew in America. Here in the States, instead of using natural colors to give it a tantalizing look, Mountain Dew is artificially colored with a petroleum-based dye called Yellow #5. You'll find the same in another landmark PepsiCo product, Gatorade. While the U.S. versions are dyed artificially with Yellow #5 and Red #40, you'll find their counterparts in Europe colored simply with black carrot juice concentrate and beta carotene (and the colors look just as vibrant and rich as they do here). Although artificial dyes are common in America, that doesn't make them okay to eat. They've been linked to several health issues, including allergies and hyperactivity in children (and may be contaminated with carcinogens). They certainly are not as safe as beta carotene and black carrot juice concentrate.

To make matters worse, PepsiCo adds brominated vegetable oil (BVO) to Mountain Dew in the U.S. but doesn't use this risky ingredient abroad. Way back in 2014, PepsiCo announced they would remove BVO from all of their American drinks following a successful petition by activist Sarah Kavanagh (who called PepsiCo out for using this additive, which is banned in Europe).[1] However, PepsiCo broke their promise and still have not removed BVO from Mountain Dew, over four years later. They already sell BVO-free Mountain Dew in other countries, so why not here?

This begs the question: Why doesn't PepsiCo just sell the same, safer, products everywhere? I'll tell ya why. It's because the U.S. food system allows companies to poison us for profit with risky additives that are banned or heavily restricted overseas. In the U.S., the government allows Big Food to largely police itself, deciding which ingredients, chemicals, and additives are "safe." As we'll see, this is a terrible policy because it leads to Americans consuming many of the very same additives and chemicals that are restricted in food in other developed countries.

This is why in Europe you don't find the artificial dyes found in American Mountain Dew, Gatorade, and most other products. You see, those dyes require a warning label in Europe. Companies don't want to slap warnings all over food packages because that wouldn't be good for business. Instead, they've found that it is more profitable to take out the offending dyes and sell a safer product in other countries. They keep selling the inferior version here because it's cheaper to produce and they can get away with it.

Do Americans care less about their health than people in other countries do? Some say so. However, I'd argue that if most Americans knew food companies are selling similar products overseas with healthier ingredients, they'd be outraged. I know I am.

I spent years investigating the differences between European and American food products, and what I found disgusted me. A college buddy of mine decided to go live in London for a few years. While she was there, I often had her go to Tesco and other European grocery stores and take pictures of the ingredient lists and send sample products to my house in the U.S. I also make it a point to look at popular products from all over the world during my travels. Comparing the same brand of products side by side but with completely different ingredient lists was maddening! The food industry has already formulated safer, better products but voluntarily sells inferior versions of these products here in America. The evidence of this runs the gamut from fast food places to boxed cake mix to cereal to candy and even oatmeal— you can't escape it. This was what really opened my eyes to how food companies exploit Americans and set me down the path of advocating for change in the food system.

MCDONALD'S SELLS *WHAT* IN LONDON?

I found the best and easiest place to look for evidence was just across "the pond" in the United Kingdom, where they enjoy some of the same types of products we do—but with totally different ingredients lists. I'm not saying that the food industry has completely eliminated their tricks abroad, but when you look at the U.K. versions of common Big Food products, they often feature fewer risky additives. It's not just the additives: I've found that many brands use less sugar and MSG overseas as well. It is appalling to witness the examples I am about to share with you.

Let's start with McDonald's. They make their iconic french fries in the U.K. with a few simple ingredients: potatoes, oil, dextrose, salt—but in the U.S. they're made with "natural beef flavor" and sodium acid pyrophosphate, and are fried in oil laced with the anti-foaming agent dimethylpolysiloxane. (McDonald's erased dimethylpolysiloxane from their online ingredients list for their fries, but its use is inconspicuously disclosed in the footer of their website—*so sneaky!*) McDonald's has found a way to cook potatoes in the United Kingdom without relying on this potentially harmful additive—and nobody seems to miss it—but they don't seem to think their American customers deserve the same benefits.

The famous fries at McDonald's are just one small example of a much bigger problem.

In the U.S., for instance, Quaker Oats sells some varieties of fruit-flavored instant oatmeal made with artificially dyed and flavored bits of dehydrated apple or figs that are manipulated with chemical additives to artificially mimic the taste and texture of the fruit indicated on the package. This includes one of their most popular flavors I used to love as a child, Quaker Strawberries & Cream, which contains no berries at all. Instead of strawberries, Quaker uses "Flavored and Colored Fruit Pieces" composed of dehydrated apples, artificial strawberry flavor, citric acid, and the artificial dye Red 40.[2] But in the U.K., they don't even attempt to sell that garbage. They instead have a product called "Oats so Simple" that has *real* strawberries in it—light-years ahead of the U.S. version that's made with artificial dyes and artificial flavors.

The ever-popular Doritos brand of chips are covered in Yellow #6, Yellow #5, and Red #40 in the U.S. and colored more simply with paprika extract and annatto in the U.K. They also sell non-GMO Doritos overseas, while the American versions have been found to have "substantial levels" of GMO corn contaminated with glyphosate weed killer.

You know what you'll find in almost every restaurant in America? Heinz Tomato Ketchup. Heinz products are GMO-free in the U.K. but are full of GMOs in the U.S. Think of that next time you're dipping your fries in ketchup!

Likewise, the most popular soft drink in America, Coca-Cola, is sweetened with GMO high-fructose corn syrup in the U.S. You won't find that in the U.K., however, where they use non-GMO cane sugar to sweeten their famous drink.

Having a premade box of flour, baking soda, and sugar all ready to go saves time when it comes to making a cake, but does saving time have to come at the expense of chemically derived and potentially toxic ingredients? The U.S. version of Betty Crocker Red Velvet Cake Mix is filled with artificial color Red #40, linked to hyperactivity in children,[3] while the same mix in the U.K. is colored naturally with paprika extract and carmine.[4] How many Americans bake this cake for their children's birthdays without knowing the risk?

We are continuously assured that our food is safe, that all those processed foods in the supermarket and items at the chain restaurants have been rigorously tested and vetted. We're told that it's foolish to worry about what's in our french fries and cake mix and sports drinks, since McDonald's and Betty Crocker and PepsiCo would never be allowed to use a dangerous additive in their foods. Or would they?

The truth is that nobody is watching out for us. When they tell you that they know their processed foods are safe, they are telling you a lie.

Food is medicine, plain and simple. If our food is sick (filled with chemicals, additives, artificial ingredients, and/or carcinogens), then collectively we as a country are going to be sick, as well.

In fact, the health of Americans is downright grim according to a report by the Institute of Medicine and the National Research Council. When compared to other countries, it declares Americans "have a long-standing pattern of poorer health that is strikingly consistent and pervasive . . . The tragedy is not that the United States is losing a contest with other countries, but that Americans are dying and suffering from illness and injury at rates that are demonstrably unnecessary."[5]

The United States spends 2.5 times more on health care than any other nation. However, when compared with 16 other developed nations, we come in dead last in terms of health and amazingly our life expectancy is decreasing for men, and near the bottom for women.[6] Here is the breakdown for you:

- More than two-thirds of United States citizens are overweight—33 percent being obese.[7]
- More than eighteen percent of children are obese.[8]

- Forty-three percent of Americans are projected to be obese in 10 years.[9]
- After smoking, obesity is America's biggest cause of premature death and is linked to 70 percent of heart disease and 80 percent of diabetes cases.

While there are many causes behind these dire statistics, undoubtedly one of the primary causes is the American diet, which is full of risky ingredients that are not used to the same extent in other countries. The food in America is overloaded with bad fats, way too much cheap refined sugar, and heaps of synthetic additives. When Big Food companies tell us that they need these ingredients, that it's not possible to remove them, or that it's too expensive, we know they're lying because they've already done it in many other countries.

The real reason the food industry doesn't remove these ingredients from their American products is because they don't care about our health, or the astronomical medical bills that are a direct result of us eating their inferior food. Instead, all they care about are their profits. Given a choice, they'll always opt for the cheaper flavor enhancer, and the cheaper color additive, and the cheaper preservative, even if these cheaper alternatives have a negative impact on our health. Government corruption and declining citizen power further prevents the food industry from making positive changes.

Big Food, of course, will tell you that the European regulators are just being overly cautious, that all of the ingredients they put in their American products are perfectly safe. After all, they've even been "approved" by the FDA. Or have they?

THE TRUTH ABOUT THE FDA

The implication is that everything allowed in processed food—preservatives, artificial sweeteners, thickeners, stabilizers, emulsifiers—has gone through some sort of rigorous testing by the FDA proving they're okay to eat. But that's absolutely not the case.

To understand why, you need a brief history of food regulation in America. Back when Congress gave the FDA authority over food additives (in 1958), there were about 800 additives.[10] Today, the number of known ingredients has swelled to about 10,000 and continues to grow.[11] Given the FDA's mission of "protecting the public health by assuring the safety, efficacy and security of . . . our nation's food supply," it would only make sense that they would be front and center in approving these new food ingredients before they hit the market; however, this is not necessarily the case. In fact, the FDA is sometimes not even aware that a new ingredient has been introduced into our food.

How is this possible?

While the FDA has approved some food additives before they hit the shelves, this has proven to be a burdensome process. The FDA claims that so as not to waste government resources, they will just let the manufacturer decide whether an ingredient is safe to eat or not.

That's right: all an ingredient manufacturer has to do is hire their own experts to claim under "reasonable certainty in the minds of competent scientists that the substance is not harmful under the intended conditions of use" and the manufacturer may deem it as "GRAS," which stands for "Generally Recognized as Safe." This is the green light to start adding it to food products.[12]

A manufacturer can voluntarily send their GRAS determination to the FDA, but this is not mandatory. Even worse, if the FDA raises questions about an ingredient received in a voluntary GRAS notice, the manufacturer can just withdraw the notice and still use the ingredient in food products! This practice is nothing short of terrifying, and allows companies to skirt around the FDA and essentially put whatever they want into our food. Since this process has been put in place, the National Resources Defense Council estimates that roughly 1,000 food chemicals have been secretly added without notification to the FDA, and say that GRAS should really stand for "Generally Recognized as Secret."[13] Even Michael Taylor, the FDA's former deputy commissioner, made the following confession: "We simply do not have the information to vouch for the safety of many of these chemicals . . . we do have questions about whether we can do what people expect of us."[14]

Simply put, you can't put your confidence in the FDA when it comes to food additives. While some additives may be safe in small quantities, the FDA cannot regulate cumulative consumption when countless additives are being added to a large number of different foods. For instance, even if you think you're eating healthfully, you could easily be eating the ingredient carrageenan (which has been linked to intestinal issues) at every meal: in your morning coffee and yogurt at breakfast, in your soup and deli-meat sandwich for lunch, and in your "diet" frozen dinner. What is the cumulative amount of carrageenan in this diet? No one is evaluating that. The FDA readily admits: "We do not know the volume of particular chemicals that are going into the food supply so we can diagnose trends. We do not know what is going on post-market."[15]

The FDA is asleep at the wheel and Big Food is in charge. The government isn't helping because no one has made it a priority for a very long time. And this isn't just my opinion. The U.S. Government Accountability Office (GAO) has called out the FDA for its lax practices and asked them to strengthen their oversight of food ingredients. The GAO's audit of the FDA in 2010 found some huge problems with the way it is running things. They found, for instance, that the FDA is not even aware of many GRAS determinations. While companies can hire their own experts to determine whether their product is safe, there are no conflict-of-interest guidelines in place. In many cases, these expert panels are composed of the "company's own staff or outside experts hired by the company." Don't you think these people might have an incentive to deliver a verdict that the company wants to hear?

The GAO also found that companies are not held accountable or required to keep records of their GRAS determinations. "The FDA has not taken certain steps to ensure companies maintain proper documentation to support their GRAS determinations," according to the report. "It [the FDA] intended to conduct random audits of data and information maintained by these companies. However, according to FDA officials, the agency has not conducted such audits." In fact, the FDA has failed to conduct ongoing reviews of GRAS substances, including those that raised concerns over 30 years ago. The GAO concluded that there are ingredients currently on the market that may not be safe: "Questions have been raised about the safety of numerous GRAS substances over the last 50 years and some have been banned as a result. In the future, other substances now considered GRAS may also prove to be unsafe."[16]

For these reasons, I believe we cannot rely on the FDA to protect us. And we certainly can't trust Big Food to self-police. After all, the food industry has consistently shown that it will only remove dangerous and unhealthy ingredients when forced to by the government, which is why the same products are healthier in the United Kingdom and Europe.

The safety of our food should be the number-one priority of the FDA. Alas, the agency often seems more concerned with helping Big Food make lots of money by using the cheapest possible ingredients and preparation methods. So the next time a food manufacturer tells us that all those chemicals and strange ingredients listed on the box are safe, that they would never be allowed to use an ingredient that was dangerous, remember this depressing truth: the safety of our food system is a lie.

ACTION STEPS: BE YOUR OWN FOOD ADVOCATE

Here's the good news: you can take matters into your own hands. Read the ingredients lists on all the packaged food you eat. If you don't recognize an ingredient, put it down and look for an alternative. By voting with our dollars in this way, we can persuade the largest food companies to change.

Even more so, join activists like me, and sign petitions and ask companies to do away with additives in their food that they don't use overseas. We have been very effective. After all, the Food Babe Army petitioned Kellogg's and General Mills and got them to remove the risky preservative BHT from many of their cereals such as Rice Krispies (they were already selling BHT-free cereals overseas). We raised awareness about the "yoga mat chemical" found in Subway's bread only in America (which they removed) and the artificial yellow dyes only in the American version of Kraft Mac & Cheese (which they also removed). We also successfully persuaded Starbucks to stop using class IV caramel color in their drinks in the U.S. (as they didn't use it overseas). These changes give me hope. I'm not optimistic that the FDA (and Congress) will ever stop being in the pocket of Big Food, but together we can work to change the American food system.

You are what you eat. You deserve food that isn't harmful.

CHAPTER 4

Weighing Calories

I have a long history with low-calorie diet food. After I got out of college, I ate a *lot* of Lean Cuisine frozen meals. I wanted quick, easy, and calorie-controlled dinners that I could eat after a long day working as a management consultant. All my girlfriends were eating them too; we'd discuss our favorite new flavors and their calorie counts. I'd pop those suckers right into the microwave, complete with their plastic wrapping, and have what I thought was a healthy, diet-friendly, ready-to-eat meal. I was convinced that my mother's traditional foods from her native country India would make me fat, and that my only hope for losing weight lay in a frozen meal with clearly marked calories and fat grams.

I also tried Smart One's frozen diet meals. They were recommended to me by a coworker who was on Weight Watchers, and they sounded like a good idea. The questionable flavor, appearance, and texture took a backseat to the meal's convenience—a couple of minutes in the microwave—and its low calorie count. With those 250 calories and 7 grams of fat, it was a personal victory in each bite.

How wrong I was. This was a period in my life when I was easily fooled by deceptive marketing and packaging. I knew nothing about real food or chemically processed ingredients. I was slowly getting sick with asthma, allergies, endometriosis, and eczema but had no idea these problems were connected to my diet. These low-calorie "diet" foods I was eating were not helping me shed the pounds either.

Sadly, way too many people still believe the diet food lies. They still think that diet foods are healthy and good for their waistlines. That fake sugar is a miracle ingredient. That the best way to lose weight is to guzzle 0-calorie soda and nosh on 100-calorie snack bars. You've heard the mantra "calories in vs. calories out"; that's what we've all been led to believe is true, right?

I confess that I fell for the calorie lie more times than I care to count. But not anymore. In the 15 years that followed, I became intimately familiar with the bleak reality of low-calorie diets—and that they are not all they're cracked up to be.

This is what I've learned.

THE TRUTH ABOUT CALORIES

Many people believe that it really doesn't matter where your calories come from; as long as you don't eat too many of them you're on the right track. However, staying thin and healthy is not this easy, or everyone would be. When planning a meal, the thought *How many calories does this contain?* rarely crosses my mind anymore. I don't count calories on a regular basis and you shouldn't have to either.

Despite what many of us have been led to believe, not all calories are equal. Your body is not going to react to 100 calories of cotton candy the same way it would to 100 calories of plain oatmeal. To further illustrate, you can eat one Twinkie loaded with high-fructose corn syrup, bleached flour, artificial colors, artificial flavors, and polysorbate 60, and it will be 135 calories. On the other hand, you can choose to eat a large pear full of fiber, phytonutrients, copper, and vitamins C and K, and still ingest about 135 calories. Which would you choose? For me, it's an easy choice, as I've learned which food will help maintain my weight and make me feel healthy and vibrant because it's giving my body the nutrients it needs to thrive.

You see, your body treats calories differently depending on the source. Dr. Dariush Mozaffarian, a medical doctor and epidemiologist, has studied how different types of foods are digested by the body and their association with weight gain. He says that although calories release the same amount of energy in a laboratory, the human body is much more complex. According to Dr. Mozaffarian in *The New York Times*, ". . . the evidence is very clear that not all calories are created equal as far as weight gain and obesity. If you're focusing on calories, you can easily be misguided."[1]

This belief has been echoed by Dr. Mark Hyman:

> It is true that, in a vacuum, all calories are the same. A thousand calories of Coke and a thousand calories of broccoli burned in a laboratory will release the same amount of energy. But all bets are off when you eat the Coke or the broccoli. These foods have to be processed by your metabolism (not a closed system). Coke and broccoli trigger very different biochemical responses in the body—different hormones, neurotransmitters and immune messengers. The Coke will spike blood sugar and insulin and disrupt neurotransmitters, leading to increased hunger and fat storage, while the thousand calories of broccoli will balance blood sugar and make you feel full, cut your appetite and increase fat burning. Same calories—profoundly different effects on your body.[2]

A recent study demonstrated that counting calories isn't the key to losing weight, and rather, the key is to eat more whole foods. Stanford researchers found that subjects who cut out processed foods and sugar, without counting calories, were able to lose significant weight. The people in the study simply focused on eating healthy whole foods and lots of vegetables, and lost a lot of weight as a result. The study's lead author, Dr. Christopher

Gardner, went on to say, "We made sure to tell everybody, regardless of which diet they were on, to go to the farmer's market, and don't buy processed convenience food crap. Also, we advised them to diet in a way that didn't make them feel hungry or deprived—otherwise it's hard to maintain the diet in the long run."[3] This just goes to show that if you're trying to lose weight, it's not about portion sizes, carbs, and fat grams. So if you're still obsessing about those things, I hope this helps you.

HOW IRONIC: SWEETENER IN DIET COKE LINKED TO WEIGHT GAIN

In 1965, the chemist James Schlatter made an accidental discovery that would transform the American diet. At the time, he was working on a drug to treat stomach ulcers. However, in the middle of one of his experiments, he licked his finger to help turn a page in his lab notebook. To his astonishment, his finger tasted astonishingly sweet.[4]

What Schlatter had discovered was aspartame, an artificial sweetener 200 times sweeter than sugar. While Americans were already familiar with saccharin—that chemical had been packaged as "Sweet'N Low" since 1957—aspartame delivered the same sweetness without the metallic aftertaste.

At first, the invention of fake sweeteners seemed like a miracle of modern food science. People could experience sweetness without the calories. Thanks to a trick of chemistry, the molecule activated our taste receptors but remained indigestible in the gut.

These diet sweeteners have since become a $1.5 billion industry: the typical coffee shop is now filled with an assortment of pastel sweetener packets of Splenda (sucralose) and NutraSweet (aspartame), while supermarkets stock hundreds of products reliant on the chemicals, from "sugar-free" candies to low-sugar yogurts. (The artificial sweetener business is also extremely profitable, since the additives are typically distilled from cheap ingredients, such as coal tar and methanol. Yum.)

On the one hand, artificial sweeteners without any calories might seem like an important tool to combat obesity. At last, we can have our cake and eat it too. And we won't gain weight!

But here's the bad news: the latest science reveals that fake sweeteners do not help us lose weight or consume fewer desserts. In fact, these sugar substitutes might increase our craving for the very substances they are supposed to replace. Put another way: the diet foods are making us fatter. Well, isn't that ironic?

The first troubling signs came from studies that examined the long-term link between artificial sweetener consumption and obesity. In a paper published in 2008, epidemiologists at the University of Texas Health Science Center followed more than 5,000 residents of San Antonio for nine years. They discovered a surprising relationship between fake sweeteners and weight gain, even after controlling for every conceivable variable. In their paper, the scientists raise the provocative possibility that artificial sweetener consumption might be "fueling—rather than fighting—our escalating obesity epidemic."[5]

Another interesting study was published in the journal *Circulation*. Researchers tracked the health condition of 9,500 men and women, ages 45 to 64, for a period of nine years. They found that the typical high-fat, sugary diet promoted metabolic syndrome and insulin resistance—both preludes to diabetes. No surprise there. But there was one shocker: the study discovered that drinking daily diet sodas full of artificial sweeteners was associated with 34 percent increased risk for metabolic syndrome, at least compared to those who didn't drink it.[6]

Of course, such data can't speak to the possible causes behind the correlation. It's entirely plausible that people who are most prone to weight gain are also the most likely to guzzle diet sodas.

However, a series of new studies—many of which look at the effects of fake sugar on the brain—raise troubling new questions about the long-term implications of consuming saccharine, aspartame, and other diet sweeteners. The first studies were led by Susan Swithers and Terry Davidson at the Ingestive Behavior Research Center at Purdue University. In a study published in

2008, the scientists fed rats yogurt sweetened either with sugar or a zero-calorie sugar substitute. When not eating the yogurt, the animals were given a standard lab pellet diet. Surprisingly, those rats fed fake sweetener consumed more calories and gained more weight.[7]

Other studies have found that animals fed sugar substitutes had slower metabolisms, displaying lower body temperatures and exercising less after ingesting sweet-tasting foods.[8] This effect exists, the researchers say, because artificial sweeteners lead to a "dysregulation" in the brain, since the presence of intense sweetness no longer signals the arrival of energy (i.e., calories). Over time, this leads the animals to lose touch with the most basic needs of the body. Instead of eating in response to hunger, they start eating all of the time. Additional research suggests that people who drink the most diet soda actually show reduced brain responses to the taste of sugar.[9] The end result is that they have to consume even more sugar—and scarf down even more calories—to experience the same amount of pleasure and satisfaction as someone who doesn't drink lots of diet soda.

These studies capture an emerging scientific consensus: fake sugars are definitely not the miracle products we were promised. Coca-Cola wants you to believe you will lose weight if you drink their diet sodas, but the truth is far more complicated. That artificial sweetener is messing with your head, making it harder for you to regulate your appetite. This is why a lot of people never reach their weight loss goals: they are constantly being pushed around by these chemical artificial sweeteners that trick the brain and body.

The negative effects of artificial sweeteners are only one example of how so-called diet foods turn out to be a big food lie. In large part, this is because the very chemicals they use to trick the tongue—to make their fake food seem real, or at least edible—are often associated with weight gain.

Take Skinny Cow ice cream sandwiches. They might seem like a responsible option—each sandwich only contains 150 calories!—but even a cursory glance at their ingredients list should make us think twice about eating them. To compensate for taking fat out of the ice cream, they bulk up the texture with a ton of additives, including corn syrup, cellulose gel, and cellulose gum. You've probably heard the bad news about corn syrup. (Hint: it's a refined form of sugar that's really bad for you.) But you might not realize that cellulose—an additive often obtained from wood by-products—has also been linked to serious digestive issues and weight gain.

For food manufacturers, cellulose is much cheaper to obtain from wood than from real food ingredients. It can be manipulated in a laboratory to form different structures (liquid, powder, and so forth) depending upon the food product it is used in.

Humans cannot digest cellulose.[10] This substance just passes through your body, while lining food industry pockets. Nice!

The gelling action of cellulose when combined with water creates an emulsion, suspending ingredients, making processed food products creamier and thicker than they would be otherwise. This is why it's a common ingredient in low-fat diet products.

While cellulose is often used to give low-fat products a creamy mouthfeel, recent research published in *Nature*, one of the most prestigious science journals in the world, highlights its potential dangers.[11] In the study, scientists at Georgia State University fed mice two of the most popular emulsifier additives used in food: polysorbate 80 and carboxymethylcellulose (aka cellulose gum, a form of cellulose). They were careful to give the animals doses equivalent to those regularly found in processed foods, such as ice cream sandwiches.

What did they find? That these common ingredients altered the makeup of the microbiome (gut bacteria) in the mice, and not in positive ways. Within days, the bacteria living in the gut of the animals showed changes consistent with increased inflammation, an underlying condition associated with many gastrointestinal disorders. And all it took was a few weeks of consuming an additive that's in most of your favorite diet foods.

What's more, these additives also induced metabolic syndrome in the poor mice: those animals exposed to the common emulsifiers had more body fat, ate roughly 20 percent more food, and had significantly higher blood sugar levels. The scientists conclude that "dietary emulsifiers may have contributed to the post-mid 20th century increased incidence of IBD [irritable bowel syndrome], metabolic syndrome, and perhaps other chronic inflammatory diseases."

So put down that Skinny Cow. Don't chug another Diet Coke. Avoid products that promise you sweetness without any calories. They're not helping you lose weight. And they might be making you ill.

Food Babe Truth Detector: The 100-Calorie Snack Fib

No doubt they're convenient, tempting, and filled with promises of self-control, but let's consider the small print on the label: salt, corn syrup, sucralose, cellulose, natural flavors, hydrogenated fat . . . this translates to highly processed and all for 100 calories.

As you dust the salty remains off your fingers, do you feel like you just ate something healthy?

I compared these snack packs ounce for ounce to the same product packaged in super-size versions, only to discover that many food companies were charging me more than twice as much for essentially the same item. This marketing ploy quickly convinced me that there are better choices that are more nutritious for the calories and a smarter use of my food dollars.

The same goes for 100-calorie products that are packaged to seem as healthy as possible. Healthy Choice Country Vegetable Soup, for instance, seems like an extremely responsible meal. The package even features brightly colored veggies! Well, if you look closely at the ingredients list, you'll soon discover that Healthy Choice soup is not such a healthy choice. While it does contain vegetables, it also contains soybean oil, added sugar, a ton of salt, and hidden MSG in the form of yeast extract. (And it also doesn't taste very good.)

Instead of overpaying for this processed soup, I like to make a big batch of Mexican lentil tortilla soup and pack it into individual portions. It's not only much better for you—it actually tastes delicious.

But maybe you don't have time to make soup. Here are some suggestions for healthy snacks that you can make yourself in virtually no time and take with you anywhere.

- Celery with organic almond butter
- Plain organic yogurt with blueberries
- A banana, large apple, or large pear
- An orange and a handful of walnuts
- A handful of frozen grapes

WHY THE LIE?

While most Americans are oblivious to it, there is a powerful industry group controlling the narrative when it comes to calories and diet foods. Many of the dollars spent to promote the belief that low-calorie processed diet foods are good for you come from the Calorie Control Council, mentioned earlier. This is a trade group of junk food and chemical companies who have banded together to fool the public about their products. Although they no longer publicize their industry members online, tax filings show the Calorie Control Council is associated with major makers of low-calorie sweeteners, such as Ajinomoto and Merisant, as well as Coca-Cola and PepsiCo.[12] To spread their message, they offer accredited educational courses to health professionals, fund research, sponsor blogs, and run several propaganda websites—including Aspartame.org and CaloriesCount.com.[13]

They engage in some undercover work to feed their lies about calories to the public. According to the Pulitzer Prize–winning organization the Center for Public Integrity, the Calorie Control Council has "a long history and a penchant for stealthy public relations tactics. The organization, which is run by an account executive with a global management and public relations firm, represents the low- and reduced-calorie food and beverage industry. But it functions more like an industry front group than a trade association."[14]

Needless to say, business is booming. The Weight Watchers Smart Ones brand alone enjoys millions in sales every year. Diet Coke outsells every other soda except for Coke itself. We spend millions more on untested diet supplements, many of which are full of caffeine and artificial sugars.

Overall, Americans are fat. The industry is banking on the assumption that we want a fast fix—and they are more than ready to sell it to us, even if it doesn't work. Just look at the stats. In 1960, about 13 percent of Americans were obese. By 2010, that percentage had nearly tripled to 37.9 percent. (Another third of us are overweight.) Nearly 8 percent of Americans are severely obese, an increase of more than 500 percent since 1960.[15]

These dire statistics help explain why, at any given time, roughly 75 million of us are on a diet. For Big Food, the diet industry is a big business opportunity, a chance to sell us more highly processed chemicals and GMO ingredients. In short, the same food industry that is making us sick has capitalized on our growing girth to make and market products that promise to alleviate the very symptoms it has created.

But they don't work. We keep getting fatter and sicker; diabetes rates are surging. Diet foods haven't solved anything.

HEALTH-WRECKING CHEMICALS IN LOW-CALORIE DIET PLANS

Recently, a friend showed me *U.S. News & World Report*'s annual ranking of its "Best Diets" in America.[16] Taking a quick glance at the list, I knew that something wasn't right. Many of the best-ranking diets rely almost solely on unhealthy, processed foods, full of additives—just like those "diet" meals I used to eat all the time in my 20s. What's more, they dissed diets that advocated eating fresh, whole foods. They've gotta be kidding, right?

When I began investigating some of these "lose weight fast" diets, I became even more outraged with what I found. This upset me because I know that most people are really trying to eat right, and these programs are feeding into desires to get the weight off as quickly as possible without considering the consequences. I came to see that these commercial diets put zero focus on the quality of the food and no care into whether the food is unprocessed, natural, organic or free of chemical additives. Although they're convenient, they're often just concoctions of health-injuring chemicals.

While slashing your calories using an out-of-the-box diet program full of low-calorie shakes, bars, and packaged meals might help you lose weight in the short term, it can be detrimental to your long-term goals. This is because the ingredients that the diet industry is packaging up for you contain risky additives that you would never cook with at home and promote an addiction to processed foods that can carry on for years.

These low-calorie products consist of dozens of chemical additives blended together with the "correct" ratios of protein, carbs, and fats, along with some synthetic vitamins and fiber mixed in to make them look healthy on the "Nutrition Facts" label. Unfortunately, the calorie count and Nutrition Facts label don't tell the real story, and you'll get a whole lot more than you bargained for when you choose to eat these foods.

Here's a rundown of some of the worst offenders:

JENNY CRAIG

This diet boasts that you can lose up to 16 pounds in four weeks, but relies almost 100 percent on processed food. This means you're sure to be eating insane amounts of preservatives and added sugar, both linked to major health risks. Jenny Craig uses some of the worst additives in their food, like carrageenan (associated with cancer and intestinal inflammation),[17] cellulose (a driver of inflammation and weight gain),[18] and the artificial sweetener sucralose (tied to leukemia and weight gain).[19]

Just look at their Philly Cheesesteak, which would definitely not pass muster in Philadelphia. The very long ingredients list reads like a greatest hits of foods to avoid. There are corn syrup solids, monoglycerides, DATEM, l-cysteine, azodicarbonamide, sodium phosphate, methylcellulose, yeast extract, dried soybean oil, caramel color, smoke flavoring, and many other chemicals that should definitely not be in your sandwich.

How could anyone call this diet healthy?

SLIMFAST

It blows my mind that this is considered an acceptable diet by anyone. On SlimFast, you knock down chemical-filled processed drinks for two of your meals, along with three of their processed snacks every day—and then you get just one home-made meal per day. You're basically gulping down tons of artificially thickened sugary drinks loaded with fake sweeteners, artificial flavors, and emulsifiers that can cause inflammation and disrupt your healthy gut bacteria. Gross.

MEDIFAST

On this diet, you eat five of its "100-calorie" products every single day, along with one home-cooked meal. The majority of the time you're eating food full of heavily processed proteins, excitotoxins, artificial thickeners and sweeteners, and synthetic vitamins and amino acids (instead of naturally occurring ones). This is nowhere near real food, which is why the Medifast Chicken Flavored Noodle Soup contains no actual chicken. (The first ingredient is "textured soy protein concentrate.") Not only is this diet severely low in calories at 800 to 1,000 calories per day on average, but it's not sustainable. Considering women are supposed to eat at the very minimum 1,200 calories per day to prevent malnutrition, the lack of calories alone on this diet is risky. Of course you'll likely lose weight when you restrict your calories to this extreme level, but what happens when you stop this diet? You guessed it. The weight pops right back up.

NUTRISYSTEM

On this diet, you eat boxed-up and processed Nutrisystem food for breakfast, lunch, and dinner. Sounds convenient! The only catch is that the meals are all filled with dozens of risky

additives, corn syrup, and hidden MSG. When you eat sweetened fake food spiked with MSG, you're falling into a trap that
spurs an addiction to unhealthy processed foods. The simple
sounding Roasted Turkey Medallions, for instance, come loaded
with mono- and diglycerides, BHA, BHT, autolyzed yeast extract,
turkey flavor, carrageenan, sodium phosphate, corn syrup, natural caramelized onion flavor, and caramel color.

Are You Filling Up on Fattening Chemicals?

There's a new foe that's thwarting our efforts to lose
weight: chemicals known as "obesogens," which are found
in foods like pesticide-sprayed fruits and everyday items like
plastic food and beverage containers.[20] So it may not just be
the triple-dip banana split that's plumping out your tummy
and hips. It may also be the plastic cup it comes in.

Obesogens are endocrine-disrupting chemicals (EDCs)
that have been linked to obesity and higher body mass index,
as well as to reproductive issues, diabetes, and cancer. Exposure to obesogens can cause your body to make more or bigger
fat cells, slow your metabolism, increase your appetite, and
decrease your satiety. How? EDCs essentially wreak havoc on
the hormones that regulate your weight.[21]

Here are the most common obesogens and how to protect
against them:

High-Fructose Corn Syrup. This is a highly sweet, chemically concocted version of corn syrup found in most processed
foods, including bread, sodas, crackers, and cookies. HFCS
influences the hormone leptin, the body's appetite switch,
increasing appetite and fat production.[22]

Hormone-Treated Dairy. Many dairy farmers inject their
animals with hormones to increase milk production. One
study that analyzed research from 10 different universities
revealed that these hormones may be associated with the obesity epidemic.

Bisphenol A (BPA) is present in many plastics and the
lining of food and beverage cans and on cash-register receipt
paper.

Tributyltin (TBT) was formerly used to preserve the bottoms of boats, which allowed TBT to leach into the water and our seafood. It's also in plastics like vinyl shower curtains. Research determined that prenatal exposure to obesogens like TBT can make you more likely to be overweight.[23]

Phthalates are plasticizers found in everything from food packaging and vinyl flooring (often in combination with TBT) to detergents, cosmetics (they help keep nail polish from cracking and hair spray flexible), air fresheners, and household cleaning products. They correlate with insulin resistance, which encourages fat storage in the body.[24]

Synthetic Pesticides, which are found in larger amounts on conventionally grown (nonorganic) produce, grains, and even in the meat of animals who feed on GMOs and conventionally grown grains.

Perfluorooctanoic Acid (PFOA) creates the nonstick surfaces on some pans and in some microwave popcorn bags, and is found in stain-resistant products. It has been shown to seep into our foods, with potentially dangerous results. A 2010 study concluded that a higher concentration of PFOA in the blood is associated with thyroid disease.[25]

What You Can Do: Limit pesticide exposure by eating organic vegetables and grass-fed meats. The conventional produce most likely to be coated in pesticides? Strawberries, spinach, nectarines, apples, grapes, peaches, cherries, pears, tomatoes, celery, potatoes, and sweet bell peppers (according to EWG's Dirty Dozen list). Choose organic grass-fed dairy. Use glass for food storage, and never heat or microwave plastic. And drink out of glass or stainless steel. Cut down on canned foods, particularly acidic ones like tomatoes, which are more apt to absorb the chemicals from the lining. Although it's challenging to avoid these things 100 percent, you'll get a health benefit by limiting exposure—and perhaps a smaller waistline.

ACTION STEPS: CHOOSE REAL FOOD FOR WEIGHT LOSS

FOCUS ON THE INGREDIENTS, NOT THE CALORIES.

As a former dedicated calorie counter, I now know how risky my old way of thinking was. When your primary concern becomes calories when looking at a food, it's far too easy to throw everything else out the window. If you're not careful, pretty soon you'll find yourself saying, "Who cares if this snack bar contains sucralose, BHT, carrageenan, and caramel color? It's only 100 calories!" That is a slippery slope that can lead to a whole host of problems much bigger than losing those last 10 pounds. So, instead of focusing on how many calories a product contains, focus on what it's really made of. The ingredients you are putting into your body are all that really matter.

GET BACK TO COOKING AT HOME.

The best solution is getting back into your kitchen and cooking real food at home, using the least processed ingredients possible. I realize this sounds old-fashioned and time consuming. But the research is clear: it's one of the best things you can do for the health of you and your family. When you cook at home, you are in complete control of the ingredients and know exactly what you're putting in your body. You'll probably notice that you don't eat as much either, as homemade food cooked from scratch is far more satisfying when it's not spiked with additives like MSG and "natural flavors" that coax you into overeating.

CHOOSE REAL, WHOLE FOODS.

Consider your gut bacteria. We've already learned that many of the emulsifiers used in popular diet foods, such as Skinny Cow ice cream sandwiches, can strip healthy bacteria from your intestinal lining. This leads to inflammation, other serious gastrointestinal illnesses, and ultimately weight gain.

However, there are reams of evidence that you can nourish your healthy gut bacteria by eating real whole foods, especially plant-based foods that are low in sugar. (Think leafy greens, vegetables, and fermented foods.) Having healthy gut bacteria is one of the keys to a healthy weight. Similar to how antibiotics (which destroy gut bacteria) are used to fatten up farm animals, it only makes sense that an unhealthy gut could fatten us up too.[26]

During my investigation into diet foods, I found an eye-opening study published in 2014 in *Annual Reviews of Public Health* that reviewed the health implications of every major diet. After looking at a vast range of data and hundreds of studies, the scientists concluded with the following advice: "A diet of minimally processed foods close to nature, predominantly plants, is decisively associated with healthy promotion and disease prevention."[27]

This seems so obvious. Yet, in the 21st century it's also a radical idea. We've been trained to associate health and losing weight with low-calorie shakes, fortified frozen foods, and dangerous supplements. When we need to lose weight, we overspend on artificial diet foods that are full of fake sugars that condition us to crave the very calories we're trying to avoid. It's a crazy downward spiral.

But the good news is that we know how to escape the spiral. All we have to do is *eat real food*. Long before I read this study, I'd been forced by my own health issues to investigate the lies of the Big Food industry. And that's when I discovered that the secret to staying in shape, feeling vital, and being healthy is eating a natural, whole food, and predominantly plant-based diet.

STAY REAL, STAY FIT

The way to create lasting change in your body is to eat food as close to nature as possible. Since I began eating this way, I have never had to diet again, and I've kept my weight off despite the challenging environment we live in with an abundance of tricky marketing, food lies, and addictive food additives.

We can't control what they are doing to our food, but we can control what we put in our mouth.

The best diet food is real food.

CHAPTER 5

Sugar: The Bittersweet Facts

Sugar seems so harmless. It's sweet, white, and everywhere: you probably have a little container of sugar on your kitchen counter, or maybe a big bag of sugar in the cupboard. Sure, the sweet crystals might give us cavities, but there's no way sugar is a dangerous ingredient. Not like fat, at least. Sugar is just energy in a delicious form, right?

Wrong. Sugar is a toxin when consumed in large quantities—and Americans are consuming sugar in massive amounts thanks to the Big Food industry. The sweet crystals wreck our health.

In order to fully understand the dangers of sugar, you first need to understand the sugar lie. And that lie begins with a 1967 article written by three Harvard scientists and published in *The New England Journal of Medicine*.[1] The academic paper looked at several different studies on the effects of sugar and fat on heart health and concluded that saturated fat was, by far, the bigger culprit. If people wanted to avoid a heart attack, the Harvard scientists said, they should avoid as much fat as possible. No eggs, steak, butter, or oils. Furthermore, they should replace these fats with more carbohydrates. Sugar was exonerated as a contributor to heart disease, while fat was crucified.

But this influential study was a lie, bought and paid for by Big Sugar. According to documents discovered by researchers at the University of California, San Francisco (UCSF), these Harvard scientists pocketed the equivalent of $50,000 (in today's dollars) from a sugar industry trade association.[2] What's worse, the sugar industry handpicked the studies to be used in the review— studies that were decidedly anti-fat and pro-sugar. Leading sugar executives even commented on early drafts, offering specific suggestions to the scientists. Since they paid for the science, they expected to get the results they wanted. And they did.

But the sugar industry didn't just pay for science that supported their toxic product—they also attacked those critics who pointed out that eating lots of sugar was terrible for the body, especially the heart. In 1972, a respected British nutritionist named John Yudkin wrote an important book that laid out the public health case against sugar.[3] The book, *Pure, White, and Deadly*, was careful and measured in tone, firmly grounded in the growing amount of scientific evidence showing that sugar—and not fat—was the leading cause of our dietary ills. Yudkin demonstrated, for instance, that:

- A person's consumption of sugar was highly correlated with heart disease.[4]

- Excess sugar is converted by the liver into fat before being released into the bloodstream.[5]

- Feeding various lab animals high-sugar diets led to a large amount of coronary plaque, even when the animals were fed a low-fat diet.[6]

Yudkin's conclusion was clear: "If only a small fraction of what we know about the effects of sugar were to be revealed in relation to any other material used as a food additive, that material would promptly be banned."[7] At the very least, we should dramatically cut back our sugar intake.

Yudkin's argument was crassly ridiculed by critics. When he struggled to publish his papers and books, Yudkin despaired that his research would ever be noticed. "Can you wonder that one sometimes becomes quite despondent about whether it is worthwhile trying to do scientific research in matters of health?" he wrote. "The results may be of great importance in helping people to avoid disease, but you then find they are being misled by propaganda designed to support commercial interests in a way you thought only existed in bad B films."[8] To make matters worse, the fierce objections to Yudkin's research discouraged other researchers from investigating the link between sugar intake and disease. The critics had won.

Needless to say, we now know (nearly 50 years later) that most of these critics were funded by the sugar industry, which was pouring money into academic studies that downplayed the link between sugar and heart disease. (As the UCSF researchers note, these tactics are very similar to those used by the tobacco industry to downplay the risk of tobacco.)

The sugar industry donated money to health organizations like the American Heart Association and American Diabetes Association, which led these groups to approve sugar as part of a healthy diet.[9] The sugar lobby even attacked John Yudkin directly, dismissing his research as "science fiction" and refusing to fund academic institutions that investigated the link between sugar and heart disease. When the sugar industry did fund research that accidentally contradicted their "sugar is healthy" stance, such as an animal study showing that sugar increased triglyceride levels in the blood and elevated the risk of cancer, they quickly pulled the plug on the project and made sure the results were never published. The end result was that the sugar industry held back nutrition science by decades.

APPETITE FOR SUGAR RAGES ON

It's hard to overstate the influence of the sugar lie. Just look at the recommended food pyramids published by the USDA. By 1992, the government was telling people to load up on 6 to 11 servings of bread, cereal, rice, pasta, and other carbohydrates and to only use fats sparingly.[10] We'd live longer if we ate more candy and fewer eggs.

The Big Food industry responded to these recommendations by developing countless low-fat, high-sugar foods. "Fat free" became an emblem of healthy eating. Never mind that most of these low-fat foods were stuffed with sugar and corn syrup.

I wish I could say that my family and I saw through these sugar lies when I was growing up in the 1980s. We didn't. Instead, we believed what the food industry told us about sugar and thought it was relatively harmless. Like most Americans, this led me to eat a lot more sugar. In fact, when I was a child I was the queen of candy! I knew every brand and every flavor, and always had candy with me. When I was low in energy, or in need of a quick snack, I treated myself to a few Runts and Starbursts. As I got older, my sugar addiction continued—well into my 20s when I'd relax on the couch with a big movie-sized box of Milk Duds. And why not? These candies were low in fat. As long I brushed my teeth afterward, I thought I'd be fine.

It turns out I wasn't alone. Americans' addiction to sugar raged for decades. By the early 1980s, the Department of Agriculture said Americans were consuming about 75 pounds of added sugars per person per year.[11] This is a whopping increase from the mere two pounds that Americans ate annually 200 years ago. (Added sugars are defined as sugars that don't come naturally from whole foods like fruits and vegetables.)

That amount had gone up to about 90 pounds per person per year by 2000.[12] By some estimates, Americans today consume roughly 152 pounds of sugar each year—which equates to 3 pounds a week.[13] Our sugar addiction has been great for business: the global sugar industry is expected to hit $100 billion in revenue by 2018, an increase of more than 25 percent over the last decade.

While our increased appetite for sugar might have brought in massive profits for the sugar industry, it was absolutely terrible for our bodies. It's not an accident that our sugar binge paralleled sharp rises in obesity and diabetes. (My father's own candy habit led to his type 2 diabetes.) In 1980, about 15 percent of Americans were obese, a rate that had been stable since 1960. Six million Americans were diabetic.[14] By 2000, when we were eating an average of 90 pounds of sugar per year, 33 percent of Americans were obese and the number of diabetics had more than doubled.[15] We blamed fat, but it was the sweet stuff's fault. Sugar did this to us.

It has become clear that sugar wreaks havoc on our bodies. The sugar lobby was able to hide the research back then, but now the evidence is undeniable. Let's take a closer look.

THE TRUTH ABOUT SUGAR

Sugar is what I think of as a "soft kill." It may not kill you today . . . but it will tomorrow, or a few years down the road. Although you might enjoy its seemingly positive effects immediately after consumption—sugar lights up the reward centers of the brain, just like an addictive drug—its detrimental effects are slowly damaging your body.[16]

Here are just a few of the negative consequences.

Weight gain. Sugar makes you gain weight by adding empty calories to your diet and jacking up your blood sugar—two processes that form excess body fat. It also screws with your appetite. According to Dr. Mark Hyman, sugar is different from other calories.[17] It scrambles all your normal appetite controls, driving your metabolism to convert it into lethal belly fat.[18] (As we've already learned in this book, all calories are not created equal.) Ditching sugar is one of the fastest and most effective ways to lose weight.

Aging. Sugar damages your skin and can lead to wrinkles. In a process called glycation, sugar molecules attach to collagen and elastin, two proteins that keep skin looking young, and create advanced glycation end products (AGEs). AGEs weaken your skin's support structure and lead to lines and wrinkles.

Inflammation. An influx of sugar in the diet increases levels of inflammatory messengers called cytokines in your body. Refined sugars processed from cane, corn, or beets, such as plain old table sugar and high-fructose corn syrup, are the baddest of the bad. These sugars have been chemically stripped of their minerals, so when you indulge in these sugars, you get zero nutrition while your body becomes more acidic, which can lead to chronic inflammation. When your body stays in a state of inflammation, you are at a greater risk of developing various diseases ranging from digestive disorders to heart disease to cancer.[19]

Liver problems. Nonalcoholic fatty liver disease (in which your liver fills with fat) now affects approximately 90 million Americans; 17 percent are children! Excessive sugar intake causes the liver to produce fat in a process called lipogenesis. The result is nonalcoholic fatty liver disease, and it puts you at risk for many other chronic diseases.[20]

Tooth decay. The sugar industry got one thing right: continually exposing your teeth to sugary foods and drinks really does erode your teeth. The bacteria naturally present in your mouth feed off sugars in your diet, producing acids that attack the enamel on your teeth and demineralizes it, eventually leading to cavities and tooth loss.

Fatigue and irritability. Added sugar makes your blood sugar go sky high—a reaction followed immediately by plummeting blood sugar. That crash and burn triggers feelings of irritability and leaves you exhausted until you get your next sugar fix. After you break the cycle of endless sugar consumption, you will no longer feel like you are living on an energy-sucking roller coaster.

Brain dangers. A study conducted by the University of New South Wales concluded that chronic sugar intake triggers changes to an area of the brain called the hippocampus, which is important for both memory and stress.[21] A UCLA study, meanwhile, found that a high-sugar diet sabotages learning and memory ability.[22] And a 2012 Mayo Clinic study found that people who eat a lot of sugar have a much higher chance of cognitive decline as they age.[23]

Poor immunity. Sugar intake weakens your immune system, so you're at a greater risk of coming down with an infection.[24] Increased insulin levels from consuming sugar also leads to high cortisol levels in the body. Cortisol is a stress hormone that further weakens your immunity.

Heart troubles. A 2015 scientific review in *Mayo Clinic Proceedings* warns that added sugar in the diet is a principal driver of "diabetes mellitus and related metabolic derangements that raise cardiovascular (CV) risk."[25] It's been shown that those who eat high-sugar diets are up to *400 percent* more likely to have a heart attack.[26]

This might sound surprising—how does this sweet white powder clog our arteries?—so it's worth spending a minute to understand how it happens. The process goes something like this: After you eat, your body secretes insulin, which helps keep your blood sugar from spiking. When you eat too much sugar, your body becomes insulin resistant, which means your pancreas has to keep pumping more insulin into the bloodstream. If your body stops responding to this insulin, you're diagnosed with type 2 diabetes. However, tens of millions of Americans are *insulin resistant*, which means their blood sugar levels are somewhat stable even as their insulin levels are chronically elevated. (This is known as metabolic syndrome.) The bad news is that those high insulin levels have many harmful effects on the cardiovascular system. In fact, recent research shows that high levels of insulin lead to high levels of triglycerides in the blood, and diminished levels of the good HDL cholesterol.[27]

It gets worse.

Research by Luc Tappy, a physiologist at the University of Lausanne, has shown that you can induce metabolic syndrome in just a few days by feeding human subjects the amount of fructose (a type of sugar) in about eight cans of soda. That's all it took. Lower doses of fructose also caused insulin resistance; it just took a few extra weeks. "There is clearly cause for immediate concern regarding potential long-term effects of very high fructose intake," Tappy writes.[28]

For decades, the sugar industry was able to con us into believing that sugar is just a tasty and convenient form of energy. Fat was the bad guy. But now we know that sugar is a "chronic toxin," and that eating large amounts of sugar for an extended period of time is just about the worst thing you can do to your diet.

WHY THE SUGAR LIE?

One word: *money.* You see, if word got out that sugar was a real health killer, the sugar industry would lose big bucks. We would ditch our beloved sweets, costing many companies a lot of business. (High-fructose corn syrup is extremely profitable, since it's distilled from GMO corn that's heavily subsidized by our government.) The industry knew that if they could get a few scientists to point the finger away from sugar, we'd focus on fat instead. This is how the sugar industry, just like Big Tobacco, spent decades paying scientists to produce papers that distracted us from the dangers of the candy aisle.

Now that we know that the true villain behind many of our health problems is sugar, the sugar industry is fighting back— with even more deceit. For instance, a recent study published in the *Annals of Internal Medicine* tried to discredit the vast amount of research showing the dangers of sugar. However, as other researchers quickly pointed out, the study was funded by an organization called the International Life Sciences Institute, a front group affiliated with Coca-Cola, Hershey's, Kellogg's, and other Big Food brands that pump up their products with lots of sugar.[29] What's more, one of the authors of the study is on the scientific board of one of the world's largest makers of corn syrup. Talk about a conflict of interest![30]

SUGAR IN "HEALTH" FOOD

It's pretty gross that the sugar industry is now copying the tactics of the tobacco industry by attempting to cast doubt on convincing health data that links sugar intake and serious health problems. What's even worse, though, is the way processed food companies have found ways to make high-sugar foods appear healthy, just like low-tar cigarettes.

Look, for instance, at the candy aisle. Today you can find candy with added vitamins, often marketed at children. Yes, vitamins in candy. We all know this does not make a piece of candy any better for you, but it is still used to reel consumers in. Companies can then compete with each other to promote their candy as healthier than the competitors'. Responsible parents don't buy gummy bears; they buy gummy bears fortified with vitamin C!

But maybe you're not a big candy fan. The sugar lobby has been so effective that it's even loaded many so-called "healthy" products—including some popular health supplements—with refined sugars like white sugar, corn syrup, high-fructose corn syrup, and artificial sugars. Vitaminwater is a good example. It contains 32 grams of sugar in a 20-ounce bottle. Most of that sugar is in the form of pure fructose too, which is like drinking a bottle of Coke. Don't let the word "vitamin" fool you.

Protein bars are another target. The Clif Builder's Protein Peanut Butter Bar might have 20 grams of protein, but it also has 22 grams of sugar. All that added sugar is disguised as beet syrup, organic brown rice syrup, and organic dried cane syrup. But all those different forms still add up to 5 teaspoons of added sugar. This is the sugar equivalent of eating two Reese's Peanut Butter Cups.

Or look at salad dressings. The very first ingredient in Brianna's Home Style Blush Wine Vinaigrette Dressing is sugar, which is why the dressing contains about 50 percent more sugar in two tablespoons (14 grams!) than a serving of Lucky Charms cereal. If you put this dressing on your salad, you are literally coating your lettuce in refined sugar.

One of the most insidious examples is a claim found on countless children's treats: "Made with Real Fruit." This could just mean that the "real fruit" is in the form of fruit juice concentrate—which is boiled-down fruit turned into a super sugary syrup. It could also include more sugar like high-fructose corn syrup and be spiked with artificial flavors and dyes. Meanwhile the big, bold marketing claim on the front of the package "Made with Real Fruit" makes you feel like you are buying something somewhat healthy and helping your child get their recommended servings of produce per day. Don't be fooled. This is nothing like grabbing an apple from the counter or some berries from the refrigerator. These products are essentially fruit by-products with everything healthy stripped out of them.

The moral of the story is that sugar is everywhere, in just about every processed food product. After all, these big food companies aren't stupid: they know that the easiest and cheapest way to make all those chemicals taste good is to coat them with various sweeteners. The end result is that roughly 80 percent of the products in the grocery store feature added sugar. Check your barbecue sauce, breads, yogurt, crackers, frozen dinners, condiments, salad dressings, pickles, cereals, and peanut butter—there's probably sugar in there! All of this has led to a completely ludicrous amount of sugar in our diets. And there's no longer any excuse for it, since the data is so clear—sugar is toxic.

THE SUGAR ADDICTION

This raises the obvious question: If sugar is so bad for us, why can't we stop eating it? When I indulged in candy, I used to hate the sugar crash, that super low-energy feeling that came an hour or so after I ate a bag of gummy worms. And yet, I'd still repeat the ritual, over and over again. I knew the candy was making me feel like crap, but I couldn't stop eating it. Why?

The answer involves the way in which large amounts of sugar can change the brain's response to sugar. According to multiple studies, people who eat lots of sweet stuff actually show reduced activity in the reward areas of the brain.[31] This means they get less pleasure from each Skittle and SweetTart. Over time, this creates a vicious cycle, since the reduced reward activity in the brain means that people need to eat even *more* sugar to get the same amount of pleasure. As a result, they develop strong cravings and seek out sweeter and sweeter foods. Before long, they're chugging Mountain Dew for breakfast. A few Skittles in the afternoon become an entire bag.

If this process sounds familiar, it's because it's very similar to what happens in the brains of drug addicts. (That's why addicts need bigger doses of the drug over time to get the same high.) As Dr. Richard Friedman writes, "The processed food industry has transformed our food into a quasi-drug . . . Their power to activate our reward circuit, rewire our brain and nudge us in the direction of compulsive consumption is unprecedented."[32]

This helps explain why so many people have tried to stop eating sugar and failed; it's a tough drug to quit. Most of us are on a sugar cravings roller coaster and don't know how to put on the brakes. Thanks to the processed food industry, we have trained the brain to crave an ingredient that's literally wrecking the body.

SUGAR-COATED RESEARCH

One of the major ways companies, organizations, government, and front groups lie to us about sugar is through shady paid-for science. As I mentioned earlier, many studies might seem convincing, but are often thinly veiled marketing ploys that undermine efforts to improve public health.

This has been going on for decades, ever since Big Sugar first attacked John Yudkin's work while simultaneously funding those skewed studies linking fat to heart disease. One of the leading scientists advocating for sugar was Frederick Stare, the chairman of the department of nutrition at Harvard. Between 1952 and 1956, the sugar industry paid for Stare and his colleagues to publish 30 papers exonerating sugar. As was noted by authors Gary Taubes and Cristin Kearns Couzens, Big Sugar even paid for a new building for the Harvard nutrition department. The single biggest donor to the building was General Foods, maker of Jell-O, Kool-Aid, and Tang.[33]

All of this money bought influence. "By the early 1970s, Stare ranked among the industry's most reliable advocates, testifying in Congress about the wholesomeness of sugar even as his department kept raking in funding from sugar producers and food and beverage giants such as Carnation, Coca-Cola, Gerber, Kellogg, and Oscar Mayer," write Taubes and Couzens. In 1975, Stare edited a white paper called "Sugar in the Diet of Man." As you can probably guess, the paper was designed to dispel the "sugar fears" of consumers and criticized those scientists who tried to link sugar to diseases such as diabetes and heart disease.[34]

The dishonesty of the Big Food lobby is why you have to become your own food truth detective. When I read about a new study, I always look to see who's funding the research, and whether or not they might have a hidden agenda (which will most likely be a profit motive). Most academic journals now require researchers to disclose any conflicts of interest in the published studies—this information typically appears at the end of the study. If the research sounds suspect to you, hunt for the original study and look for this notation. *Follow the money.*

Of course, conflicts of interest aren't always listed honestly, even in prominent journals. In many cases, I've been forced to look up which boards the scientists serve on and who has paid them to be a consultant. (If they've received consulting fees from processed food companies, you can probably guess what their research will show.) I recommend that when you read a study that seems suspect, you look extra carefully at the sources of funding. We've been duped by the sugar lobby for long enough.

You might not think this tainted research can have a big impact on your diet, but you'd be wrong. Just look at Gatorade. As was noted in the *British Medical Journal*,[35] PepsiCo and Coca-Cola have spent millions of dollars looking into the "science" of dehydration in order to trick people into drinking sports drinks like Gatorade and Powerade. (There's even a Gatorade Sports Science Institute.) One of their greatest cons was producing research showing the beneficial effects of these drinks— research that just happened to be produced by scientists on their payroll. When the *British Medical Journal* looked in detail at these studies, they concluded that less than 3 percent of them were valid. The rest were tainted by major scientific and statistical errors.

Nevertheless, such science has led generations of athletes to conclude that they'll run faster and perform better if they guzzle a neon-colored sports drink full of sugar and artificial ingredients. (My parents always bought me Gatorade when I was sick; orange was my favorite flavor.) But the shoddy science has led us astray: Gatorade isn't helping, or even staving off dehydration. If it's doing anything, it's triggering a dangerous cycle of inflammation that will make workout recovery more difficult.

Still not convinced that the lies of the sugar industry shape the way we think about sweets? Here are a few more recent examples that, if they weren't such clear evidence of the sugar industry's collusion with scientists, would make you roll over in laughter. And this stuff isn't happening in the distant past. This is happening right now. We're *still* being lied to.

Thin Kids and Candy. When I read the following headline— "Does candy keep kids from getting fat?"—I went nuts. If this were true, it would be a shocking scientific finding, especially since it would contradict decades of research into the hazards of candy (and also contradict common sense!).

But this shocking finding was full of holes. The study that inspired such an egregious headline was funded by none other than a candy trade association. As can be expected, the researchers were serving the interests of the candy makers they were working for. Their research was based on government surveys that asked people to recall what they had eaten in the past 24 hours. The problem with this methodology is that people often don't remember what they ate, which is what led the researchers to admit that their data "may not reflect usual intake" and "cause and effect associations cannot be drawn."[36] Translation: the results were pretty much bogus. The thinner-children-eat-candy message sure generates headlines, but what a load of crap. If you want to quickly pack on a few pounds and get chronically sick, eat lots of candy and refined sugar.

The Chocolate Milk Cure? Companies will use any "research" tactic necessary to market products and boost sales. One of the most egregious examples of this involved a small chocolate milk company called Fifth Quarter Fresh and a University of Maryland study it paid for. The company wanted publicity touting the ability of its chocolate milk to help high school athletes recover from concussions—publicity that would coincide with the Will Smith movie *Concussion*, according to e-mails obtained by the Associated Press.[37] The whole effort was suspect because the actual study findings weren't even made available. Fortunately, the university conducted an internal investigation, disavowed the study, and returned the research funds to Fifth Quarter.

Ice Cream for Breakfast Makes You Smarter. Huh? Here's a story that went viral: A website in Japan (Excite.co.jp) published a story making this exact claim. As was reported by *Business Insider*, "According to Excite, Koga found that people who ate ice cream had faster response times and more brainwave activity than those who had more normal breakfasts. This, apparently, is evidence for ice cream's brain-boosting powers." The article cited a single study from Kyorin University, funded by an unnamed sugar company. Sure, maybe a high-glucose meal like ice cream will perk you up—temporarily—but if you do this every morning you'll soon wreck your health. Your mother was right: ice cream is not a good breakfast food.[38]

Processed Cereals Help You Lose Weight. I've always loved cereal. As a child I downed bowls of sugary Golden Grahams for breakfast. (I sometimes ate them for dinner too.) Thankfully, I found much healthier cereal later in life. But before I tell you about my favorite kinds (see Chapter 9), we must discuss how the cereal giants use paid research to tout the "health" of their sugary products.

Way back in the 1990s, you'd find claims on boxes of Kellogg's Special K cereal that a recent study found that adding breakfast to your routine could help you lose weight. The backing for this claim? A study funded by Kellogg's (but you wouldn't find their backing of the study disclosed on the box). As the AP reported, "That was the little piece they put on the cereal box," said David Schlundt, a coauthor of the study of about 50 women. Not mentioned on those boxes: Regular breakfast eaters who started skipping the meal lost even more weight, compared to those who stuck with their routines.[39] You wouldn't believe a study on cigarettes that was funded by Philip Morris, and you probably shouldn't believe a study on cereal paid for by a company whose bottom line depends on Froot Loops, Apple Jacks, and Frosted Flakes.

When I read studies like this, I remember that statistics are easy to manipulate, especially when you know what result you're looking for. Instead of being distracted by the latest clickbait headline and health claims made by food companies, it's important to focus on the vast body of evidence showing that refined sugars are bad for us. And most breakfast cereals are full of exactly that. According to a report by the Environmental Working Group, children's cereals contain, on average, 34 percent sugar. After analyzing 1,556 cereals on the U.S. market, the group discovered that 92 percent of cold cereals in the U.S. are preloaded with added sugars, and every single cereal marketed to kids contains added sugar.[40]

Skittles as Cattle Feed? No, this is not a joke from late-night TV. For many years, cattle have been getting their carbs from "rejects" set aside by bakeries and candy makers. In 2012, CNN reported that when the price of corn is on the rise, cheap treats like Skittles become even more appealing to farmers. As you can probably guess, the candy is very effective at fattening up the animals.[41]

Should we be worried that cows are eating too much sugar? Not if you listen to some farmers and animal nutritionists. They claim that as long as the cows are getting the right ratio of carbs, protein, vitamins, and minerals, it does not matter if it's coming from corn or candy. Really? I just feel sorry for the poor animals. Their bodies certainly weren't designed to handle so much sugar.

But then neither were ours.

THE LIE LIVES ON

In 2016, the USDA released its updated Dietary Guidelines for Americans, with a focus on preventing type 2 diabetes, hypertension, and heart disease. This report officially recommended that we should consume less than 10 percent of our calories from added sugars.[42]

When I read these guidelines, I began thinking about what that sugar recommendation means for a typical person. I did a little research, so let's look at the following scenario.

Suppose you eat around 2,000 calories a day. If you get 10 percent of your calories from added sugar, you're eating 200 calories of unnecessary sugar every day. Because sugar has 4 calories per gram, that's equivalent to about 50 grams of sugar per day, or about 12 teaspoons. (There are about 4.2 grams of sugar in a teaspoon.) That's about the same amount of sugar that's in a can of soda and a Twinkie.

Is it okay to eat that much sugar each day? I don't think so. The science has come a long way in the last few decades, but the sad truth is that our diets haven't caught up with the data: we're still eating way too much of the sweet stuff. It's time to stop.

Food Babe Truth Detector

Our own FDA has allowed a version of high-fructose corn syrup to go by the name of "fructose" in food products! HFCS is a sweetener that the food industry loves to use because it's much cheaper than real sugar and helps preserve their products so they can sit on the shelf for a long time. Not only is HFCS generally made from GMO corn, but one study found that it can be contaminated with toxic mercury. HFCS has been shown to contribute to type 2 diabetes, especially in children, and this is why I consider it to be one of the top sweeteners to avoid. HFCS-90 is a variation of high-fructose corn syrup that contains way more fructose than regular HFCS. When HFCS-90 is used, the ingredient label won't indicate that high-fructose corn syrup is an ingredient; rather, it can be deceptively listed as simply "fructose" or "fructose syrup" without any reference to corn syrup.[43] Regular HFCS contains up to 55 percent fructose, whereas HFCS-90 has 90 percent fructose by weight. That's nine times more fructose than the average fruit!

How sneaky is that? Don't be fooled!

Are You Hooked on Sugar?

Answer these 15 questions to find out.

1. Do you experience a high, excitement, or sense of relief when you eat sweets?
   - ❏ Yes
   - ❏ No

2. Do you reach for sweets when you're stressed out or having a bad day?
   - ❏ Yes
   - ❏ No

3. Do you often go out of your way to buy sweets?
   - ❏ Yes
   - ❏ No

4. Have you ever eaten sugary foods in secret?
   - ❏ Yes
   - ❏ No

5. Do you often feel guilty after eating sweets?
   - ❏ Yes
   - ❏ No

6. Do you routinely eat sweets when you're alone?
   - ❏ Yes
   - ❏ No

7. Do you find yourself often dwelling on which sweets you'll eat next?
   - ❏ Yes
   - ❏ No

8. Does your energy drop after you eat a lot of sweets?
   - ❏ Yes
   - ❏ No

9. Do you worry that the amount of sugar you eat will harm your health, but you keep eating it anyway?
   - ❏ Yes
   - ❏ No

10. Would you, someone in your family, or some friends describe you as having a sweet tooth?
    - ❏ Yes
    - ❏ No

11. If you were alone with a box or package of sweets, would you eat the whole thing?
    - ❏ Yes
    - ❏ No

12. Do you eat or drink sugary foods or beverages (including those made with artificial sweeteners) every day?
    - ❏ Yes
    - ❏ No

13. Do you need to drink your coffee or tea with sugar or a sweetener?
    - ❏ Yes
    - ❏ No

14. Do you often feel powerless when tempted by something sweet?
    - ❏ Yes
    - ❏ No

15. After indulging, do you promise yourself you will swear off sweets?
    - ❏ Yes
    - ❏ No

Scoring: Like most people, you may have a healthy relationship with sweets, and they don't rule your life. If you answered "yes" to five or more questions, your sweet tooth may be strong. Consider scaling back on your sugar intake (see my action steps below). A growing amount of research is showing that added sugar is more injurious to health than was previously believed.

ACTION STEPS: KICK YOUR SUGAR HABIT

For me, sweets are one of those guilty pleasures that I enjoy after dinner or on special occasions—and let's face it; those special occasions seem to pop up all the time. What makes a sugar habit even harder to kick is that sugar is everywhere, often hiding in foods that are supposed to be good for you. Nevertheless, this is one bad habit worth kicking: sugar is so toxic in large amounts that giving it up just might change your life. Here's how to do it:

EAT AT A REGULAR TIME EVERY DAY.

By skipping meals or going for a long period of time between meals, you're setting yourself up for disaster. Instead of having the needed energy to make healthier choices, you'll seek out whatever is quick and easy. This often leads to eating more processed foods in larger quantities. Let me interject here that you must rid your home of these foods—and all sugary foods. So start eating healthy meals at the exact same time each day, and your body will sing.

BALANCE YOUR MEALS.

Include plenty of whole foods that contain healthy fats and protein. Eat lots of greens too, because they're loaded with phytonutrients that keep you feeling well and energetic.

INTRODUCE HEALTHY FATS.

By adding healthy fats into your diet, you'll feel full longer—a situation that will reduce cravings and promote weight loss. Some of my favorite healthy fats are avocados, coconut oil, cold-pressed oils, nut and seed butters, organic lean meat, wild-caught fish, flaxseeds, chia seeds, and hemp seeds.

58 Different Names for Sugar

Below are some words to watch for on labels when trying to limit added sugars in your diet.

Agave nectar	Glucose
Barbados sugar	Glucose solids
Barley malt	Golden sugar
Beet sugar	Golden syrup
Blackstrap molasses	Granulated sugar
Brown sugar	Grape sugar
Buttered syrup	High-fructose corn syrup
Cane juice crystals	Honey
Cane sugar	Icing sugar
Caramel	Invert sugar
Carob syrup	Lactose
Castor sugar	Malt syrup
Confectioner's sugar	Maltodextrin
Corn syrup	Maltose
Corn syrup solids	Maple syrup
Crystalline fructose	Molasses
Date sugar	Muscovado sugar
Demerara sugar	Raw sugar
Dextrane	Refiner's sugar
Dextrose	Rice syrup
Diastase	Sorbitol
Diastatic malt	Sorghum syrup
Ethyl maltol	Sucrose
Evaporated cane juice	Sugar
Fructose	Syrup
Fruit juice	Treacle
Fruit juice concentrate	Turbinado sugar
Galactose	Yellow sugar

USE SPICES.

Add naturally sweet spices to foods when you have a craving for something sweet. For example, cinnamon on oatmeal can replace actual sugar and taste just as wonderful.

DRINK PLENTY OF WATER.

Some people mistake dehydration for a sugar craving. Try drinking an eight-ounce glass of water and waiting 10 to 15 minutes before eating. You can also slice some fresh fruit like lemons, limes, oranges, or cucumber into the water for a burst of sweet flavor.

TAKE YOUR MIND OFF CRAVINGS WITH EXERCISE.

When the urge to splurge on something sugary hits, start moving. The simple act of focusing your mind on a different activity will fight off cravings. That's because it is usually when your mind is idle that you start thinking about food. Take back your power with exercise. It releases feel-good endorphins that can provide a high similar to that of sugar or junk food, only this high isn't followed by a sudden crash. Not only will you feel better about yourself and the decision you made, but you are also creating a new healthy habit.

ENJOY FERMENTED FOODS.

I've found this to be one of the best ways to fight cravings. Fermented foods include but are not limited to: yogurt, kimchi, sauerkraut, miso, and apple cider vinegar. They banish stubborn sugar cravings as well as adding healthy bacteria to your gut. Those healthy bacteria actually eliminate excess sugar because they feed on it.

BOOST SEROTONIN LEVELS NATURALLY.

You can do this easily by making sure you're getting enough sleep each night. When your body has ample time to recharge, you may find that your sugar cravings aren't as intense.

Use fruit to satisfy a sugar craving.

Fresh whole fruits contain natural sugar along with fiber—a combo that helps reduce spikes in blood sugar. So grab fresh fruit when sugar cravings come on, and you'll kill the craving. Plus, fresh fruit supplies vitamins and antioxidants, which you can't get from cookies or cake.

Avoid using artificial sugar substitutes.

Please do not reach for Splenda, Equal, Sweet'N Low, or other low-calorie sugar sweeteners with their false promises. They will only create real cravings for real sugars. (More on that in Chapter 5.) After you've been off sugar for a few weeks, introduce small amounts of natural sweeteners back into your diet. These include dates, coconut sugar, honey, maple syrup, or stevia.

The good news is that if you give your body a break from sugar, you'll eventually develop a distaste for very sweet foods. The reward areas of your brain will reset and those cravings for sickly sweet products will disappear. What's more, you'll naturally eat less sugar in the long run because your body is getting real nutrition from food that hasn't been chemically altered. What a wonderful habit to develop and keep for life!

I know that giving up sugar can feel impossible, especially in a world where every supermarket aisle is filled with excessively sweet products. But the truth is that we can survive without added sugar. In fact, all of the sugar our bodies need is present in the naturally healthy fruits and veggies we eat every day. So join with me and promise to never fall for the food industry's biggest con: sugar is not a healthy part of your diet. It's not a harmless source of energy or a tasty treat.

It's a chronic toxin and should be treated as such.

CHAPTER 6

Sipping Sabotage

One of the top three food companies in the world is Coca-Cola. Do you see what's wrong with that picture? The majority of what they produce isn't even real food—it's a sugar-laden drink full of processed additives. They have enormous power in the marketplace and have used their influence to infiltrate our every move about nutrition and health. They drive the conversation in the media, are at the table when government policies are made, and pay academics under the table to promote their agenda.

You could say my fight against Big Soda really began in a Starbucks. A few years ago, it was Pumpkin Spice Latte season, and I couldn't help but notice that just about everyone seemed to be enjoying this incredibly sweet dessert masquerading as a coffee drink. In fact, the Pumpkin Spice Latte is Starbucks's most popular seasonal drink—they sell millions every year. Almost everyone has had one, and you might have had a few yourself.

The popularity of the drink led to several readers e-mailing me about the ingredients. They wanted to know what, exactly, was in all those syrups, powders, and sauces used to make the drink.

So I did the obvious thing: I e-mailed Starbucks asking for the complete list of ingredients in the Pumpkin Spice Latte. This is the response I got:

"The Pumpkin Spice Latte is of pumpkin and traditional fall spice flavors combined with espresso and steamed milk, topped with whipped cream and pumpkin pie spice. If you ever have any questions or concerns in the future, please don't hesitate to get in touch."

I hate when companies are condescending. Starbucks was pretending to answer my questions while totally avoiding the truth. What's in that whipped cream? Is it just cream and sugar? (Almost certainly not.) And what about that "pumpkin pie spice"? If it's so wholesome and natural, why not just tell us the actual ingredients? My radar went up because they were being so evasive. After several more e-mails back and forth, they were still refusing to tell me what was in the drink:

"While we understand that some customers would like to know the nutrition information for their specific customized beverage, unfortunately we are unable to provide this level of detail for every beverage customization request. The beverage information that is available on Starbucks.com reflects the beverage offerings currently on our menu with the most common customization options."[1]

I found this outrageous. I strongly believe that we have a right to know what's in the food we eat. Starbucks likes to brag about its transparency, but they refused to tell us what they put into their lattes. What were they trying to hide?

This meant I had to take matters into my own hands. I began by persuading a barista at my local Starbucks to let me look at their various drink components. Despite the assurances of corporate headquarters, the Pumpkin Spice Latte wasn't just espresso, syrup, and steamed milk. I eventually uncovered the complete ingredients list (as it was at the time):

Milk, espresso (water, brewed espresso coffee), pumpkin spice flavored sauce (sugar, condensed nonfat milk, high fructose corn syrup or sweetened condensed nonfat

milk [milk, sugar], annatto [for color], natural and artificial flavors, caramel color [class IV], salt, potassium
sorbate [preservative]), whip cream (whipping cream,
Starbucks vanilla syrup [sugar, water, natural flavors,
potassium sorbate, citric acid, caramel color {class IV}]),
pumpkin spice topping: cinnamon, ginger, nutmeg,
clove, sulfites.

And that's when I finally understood why Starbucks took
such pains to hide their ingredients—they didn't want their
customers to know about the risky additives in their best-selling
items. (Especially that innocuous sounding caramel color.)

Case in point: if you ordered the Pumpkin Spice Latte,
you'd get two doses of class IV caramel coloring, one dose in
the syrup and another in the whipped cream. Let me explain
why this particular caramel color is so troubling. There are four
different types (classes) of caramel coloring. The type used by
Starbucks (class IV) is manufactured by heating ammonia and
sulfites under high pressure, which creates carcinogenic compounds, notably the dangerous substance 4-methylimidazole
(4-MEI). One study funded by the U.S. government found that
feeding mice caramel coloring IV (which contained 4-MEI)
increased their risk of developing lung cancer and leukemia.[2]
The International Agency for Research on Cancer, a widely
respected division of the World Health Organization, classifies
4-MEI as "possibly carcinogenic to humans."[3] Furthermore,
an investigation by *Consumer Reports* found excessive levels
of 4-MEI in many popular U.S. drinks.[4] They didn't test the
Pumpkin Spice Latte, probably because they didn't realize Starbucks used this coloring. I mean, why would you need to color
coffee brown?

After confirming the use of class IV caramel coloring in
the Pumpkin Spice Latte, I wrote a blog post exposing this on
foodbabe.com. The piece quickly went absolutely viral with over
10 million views in 2014. Within days, major news outlets had
picked up the story. I appeared on a popular national TV morning show to discuss my findings.[5]

It wasn't long before I heard back from Starbucks. After a few months, I received what I had been waiting for. A representative told me that Starbucks was now in the process of transitioning to a new formula, which is free from caramel coloring.[6] They were also going to post drink ingredients on their website. Success! Needless to say, I was delighted to hear that our collective activism had managed to get rid of a dangerous ingredient from an extremely popular drink and that we would finally get true transparency out of Starbucks. This was a major victory for us— and a major defeat for the industry that creates caramel coloring and the Big Soda brands who depend on caramel color to make their products look appealing. As you will see in this chapter, this was a big threat to the soda industry's profits.

We have already learned about the toxic effects of sugar and the dangerous food lies the sugar industry has perpetuated for decades. Now we will focus on the evils of soda and the lies of the soda industry, who have tried for decades to defend a food that has zero nutritional value and is loaded up with toxic ingredients. Long story short: there is no mass-produced food product that has been worse for the health of Americans. If we got rid of soda, we'd all live healthier and longer lives.

That's why they spend so much on feeding us lies.

THE TRUTH ABOUT SODA

I probably don't need to tell you that soda isn't healthy. Almost everyone knows this. However, consumers often don't realize just how hazardous soda really is. When you drink soda, you're ingesting a concentrated slurry of sugar and controversial chemicals that screw with the most basic processes of your body.

As the Centers for Disease Control notes, soda consumption is associated with a long list of health problems, including obesity, type 2 diabetes, heart disease, kidney disease, fatty liver disease, gout, and even asthma.[7] (Good luck finding a major internal organ that is *not* harmed by excessive soda consumption.) The more soda you drink, the more likely you are to suffer from these diseases, strongly suggesting that high levels of soda consumption play a causal role. But even moderate consumption of soda can put you at risk. A long-term study composed of nearly 90,000 women found that drinking more than two sugary drinks a day increased risk of heart attack or heart disease deaths by 40 percent compared to women who rarely indulged in sugary drinks.[8] Another study found a 20 percent increased risk of heart attack if you drank just a single 12-ounce soda per day.[9]

The primary aspect making soda so dangerous is that the drinks contain a huge amount of sugar without any fiber. When you eat a piece of fruit, you might also get a significant amount of sugar. (A big apple can contain up to 18 grams.) But this sugar comes along with fiber, which slows down the release of that sugar into the bloodstream. There is no sudden spike.

But sodas have no fiber. As a result, they overwhelm our internal organs with sweet stuff, sending the pancreas and liver into overdrive. That excess sugar is then converted into fatty globules in the bloodstream, which can lead to heart disease. What's more, the lack of fiber means that the empty calories in soda don't leave us feeling satisfied, which can cause us to eat more than we should, or even drink another soda. And if that wasn't bad enough, sodas are also loaded with dangerous preservatives like phosphoric acid.

So maybe you don't drink regular soda. That's good.

In my experience, however, many people replace these sugary beverages with other drinks from the soda industry that they think are healthier. Coca-Cola doesn't just make Diet Coke sweetened with aspartame—they also make Coke Zero Sugar (sweetened with aspartame and the zero-calorie artificial sweetener acesulfame potassium [Ace-K]), Coke Life and an array of Diet Coke flavors, from Mango to Blood Orange. (In actuality, these new Diet Coke "flavors" are really nothing more than old Diet Coke with a new flavor added and a slick marketing campaign.)

And then we've got flavored waters flooding the market. These fruity waters and fizzy "sugar free" drinks are being promoted as healthy alternatives to regular Coke, Pepsi, and Sprite. But are they actually good for us?

If they seem too good to be true, that's because they are. Most of these zero-calorie alternatives are filled with controversial additives that can sabotage your weight and your health— even if they have little added sugar, look like bottled water, or have really short ingredients lists.

Let's start with their main selling point, which is that they have zero calories. In many cases, the lack of calories is because they are artificially sweetened with sucralose. Sucralose (which goes by the brand name Splenda) is created by chlorinating sugar in a lab, and while it may be insanely sweet and have no calories, it's also linked to cancer. In 2016, the Center for Science in the Public Interest downgraded their rating of sucralose from "caution" to "avoid" after a study came out linking the sweetener to leukemia and related blood cancers in male mice.[10]

Artificial dyes in these drinks (like Yellow #5, Red #40, and Blue #1) are derived from petroleum and linked to several health issues, including allergies, cancer, and hyperactivity in children.[11] If that's not bad enough, these drinks can be preserved with potassium benzoate, which can form the carcinogen benzene when combined with vitamin C (which is present in many of the drink flavors).[12] That's a dangerous chemical cocktail in a plastic bottle.

The sheer awfulness of soda should make us wonder why we buy so much of the stuff. The statistics are staggering: roughly 63 percent of U.S. children drink at least one soda per day, while about 30 percent drink two or more. This comes as no surprise, as 60 percent of schools sell them. On average, American adults consume 145 calories from sugary beverages each day.

How is this possible? How do Coke and Pepsi still rack up billions in sales, even when we know that their products can dramatically increase the risk of serious illnesses like type 2 diabetes and heart disease? Why are there still entire aisles dedicated to these toxic drinks in most grocery stores?

The answer to these questions brings us to the terrible soda lie.

THE SODA LIE: YOU'RE JUST LAZY

Soda companies such as Coke and Pepsi—along with their friends at the American Beverage Association (the main soda trade association) and International Life Sciences Institute (a front group partially sponsored by Coca-Cola)—have focused on telling one very big lie. According to Big Soda, we get fat because we don't exercise enough, not because we eat or drink too much sugar.

Coca-Cola summarizes this idea on its website: "There is increasing concern about overweight and obesity worldwide, and while there are many factors involved, the fundamental cause in most cases is an imbalance between calories consumed and calories expended. Our goal is to help people around the globe understand the importance of a sensible, balanced diet and the health benefits from increasing their levels of physical activity."[13] In other words, you need to work out more to avoid obesity (but keep drinking that Coke!).

This approach makes perfect sense for Coke, at least from a business perspective. Since they make their money by filling us up with empty calories, it's only logical that they would try to focus attention on increased exercise. (Especially if that leads us to drink more Powerade and Vitaminwater, both of which are owned by Coca-Cola.) In 2012 Coca-Cola published their very own "Work It Out" calorie calculator, an app that would calculate how much you needed to exercise to burn off that Coke you just drank. This focus on calories in, calories out also allows Coke to vigorously push its low-calorie beverages to persuade dieters to keep drinking Coca-Cola products. But here's the truth: as we explored in Chapter 4, not all calories are equal—especially when they consist of refined sugar and natural flavors that increase food cravings.

This is faulty logic and illustrates Coke's attempt to shift the blame on obesity from sugar consumption to lack of physical activity. If you're fat and drink lots of soda, the problem isn't soda; it's that you're *lazy*. This contradicts dozens of well-done studies showing that, for the vast majority of people, exercise is not an effective weight loss tool. Exercise is still really good for you, but if you're looking to shed pounds, you probably need to change your diet, not join the gym.

The fact that Coca-Cola and other food industry giants are getting away with this orchestrated deception is unbelievable. They've helped create the obesity crisis. Now they're trying to deflect blame—blaming us for being lazy instead—while simultaneously peddling a new generation of unsafe low-calorie drinks.

How stupid do they think we are?

WHY THE LIE?

Big Soda will do anything to keep and grow its market share of soft drinks. In fact, Big Soda's tactics have frequently been compared to those of the tobacco industry.

From the 1950s until the late 1990s, the tobacco industry orchestrated an elaborate campaign of disinformation to discredit the science connecting cigarettes to lung cancer and other diseases. Today, the soda industry is engaged in its own campaign of disinformation to cast doubt on the science linking sugar-sweetened beverages to negative health consequences.

And they're telling the lies with help from people we should be able to trust for health information, such as dietitians, academics, trade groups, the government, and others.

Need proof? Take a look.

Big Soda, Big Spenders. In 2016, the trade group for Big Soda compensated a group of dietitians to use Twitter to tweet against soda taxes, saying such things as "Soda taxes fall flat" and "Better-informed consumers, not taxes, can help prevent obesity."[14] These dietitians are supposed to be experts offering advice on healthy eating, but instead they are shilling for Big Soda's political gain. Isn't that crazy?

Around the country since 2009, Big Soda's three reigning members—the American Beverage Association, Coca-Cola, and PepsiCo—have disbursed around $67 million to defeat soda taxes and fight warning labels regarding added sugar, according to the Center for Science in the Public Interest.[15] That much money buys a lot of influence. So the next time you see a supposed expert telling us that soda isn't so bad, your next question should be whether they're on the payroll of the soda industry.

A Bubbling Conflict of Interest. Big Soda has helped fund nearly 100 medical and public health organizations, according to a report published in the *American Journal of Preventive Medicine*.[16] Those organizations have included the American Diabetes Association, the American Heart Association, and the American Academy of Pediatrics. These are groups that are supposed to support public health. Many of these organizations have a direct mission to fight obesity, yet they have taken money from soda companies.

Naturally, this is a huge conflict of interest. How can the American Diabetes Association accept big bucks from a soda company when there is clear proof that soda is helping drive the huge increase in type 2 diabetes? They are taking money from the very companies that are contributing to the problem they are trying to solve.

Coke Fights Obesity? The Coca-Cola Company was instrumental in shaping and funding a nonprofit group called the Global Energy Balance Network, led by a professor at the University of Colorado School of Medicine.[17] The group's mission? To combat obesity!

The group received $1.5 million from Coke (and asserted the funds didn't influence their work). Yet e-mails obtained by the Associated Press told a different story. Coke had a hand in selecting the group's leaders, along with the content and videos that it put out. According to the AP, "the group would use social media and run a political-style campaign to counter the 'shrill rhetoric' of 'public health extremists' who want to tax or limit foods they deem unhealthy."[18] Even worse, internal e-mails reveal the soda company had high hopes it would "quickly establish itself as the place the media goes to for comment on any obesity issue." As was uncovered in a recent paper in *Journal of Epidemiology and Community Health*, internal documents from the company reveal that they saw the front group as a "'weapon' to 'change the conversation' about obesity amidst a 'growing war between the public health community and private industry.'"[19]

They disbanded in late 2015 after the e-mails surfaced that exposed Coke's efforts. Coke stopped working with the group and informed the AP it had accepted the retirement of their chief health and science officer, Rhona Applebaum. And yet, the damage had been done, as the front group had succeeded in confusing millions of consumers about the dangers of soda and sugar. This fiasco is just one recent example how far Big Soda will go to protect their profits.

Pouring Money into Experts. In 2015, *The New York Times* exposed that Coke had provided millions of dollars in funding to fitness and nutrition experts to discredit the link between sugary drinks (like soda) and obesity, while suggesting Coke as a healthy treat.[20] (Coke also funds nutritionists who push junk food in general—they had one professor on the corporate payroll who said he lost 27 pounds eating Twinkies.)[21] Several dietitians, paid by Coke, wrote online pieces and appeared on morning news programs advising consumers to enjoy a mini-can of Coke or small soda as a snack. Positioning Coke as a healthy snack is a total joke. But I'm not laughing.

The money keeps flowing. Coke acknowledged that they have paid $2.1 million directly to health experts. In addition, they've invested $21.8 million in pro–soft drink research. Of these health experts working on Coca-Cola's dime: 57 percent were dietitians, 20 percent were academics, and the remaining experts were primarily doctors, fitness experts, authors, and chefs.[22]

The CDC. The Centers for Disease Control and Prevention (CDC) is a federal agency charged with improving public health in the U.S. It turns out this agency was in bed with Coke for years. This became apparent in June 2106, when Carey Gillam at U.S. Right to Know broke the story that a high-ranking official at the CDC, Dr. Barbara Bowman, had been in regular communications with top Coca-Cola advocate Alex Malaspina, a former Coca-Cola executive and founder of the front group

International Life Sciences Institute (ILSI), which is partially sponsored by Coke. Dr. Bowman left the CDC a mere two days after damaging e-mails between the two were exposed, revealing that she had been providing guidance to him on how to influence beverage and sugar policy at the World Health Organization. Additional e-mails showed close communications between another senior official at the CDC, Michael Pratt, and ILSI. In another role, Pratt is a professor at Emory University, which credits Coca-Cola as a huge financial supporter. So much so that Emory jokes it's "unofficially considered poor school spirit to drink other soda brands on campus."[23]

Junking Up the FDA. In the same e-mails exposing the CDC, more details emerged about this friend of Coca-Cola who has been quietly campaigning our government officials to support Big Soda. Alex Malaspina, who at one time was able to infiltrate the World Health Organization with industry-friendly scientists, money, and research, has more recently set his sights on the U.S. Food and Drug Administration with a campaign to discredit food industry critics like myself.

The year following our campaign to get "yoga mat" out of Subway and my viral post about the caramel coloring in the Pumpkin Spice Latte, Coca-Cola took aim at our ability to convince major food companies to remove additives from their products. At the coaxing of his friends over at Coca-Cola, Alex Malaspina sent a private e-mail to Michael Taylor, a top FDA head, proposing the FDA hold a roundtable discussion on "Junk Science Reporting and Its Unintended Consequences." What gave rise to such a suggestion? As Coca-Cola put it in their proposal: "Recent events—the vaccine scare in California, investigations by AMA and others into Dr. Oz, criticism of the Food Babe's misuse of science and pledges by food service establishments and companies to remove ingredients in response to 'consumer pressure'—have created a window of opportunity to drive an important message about the pervasiveness of pseudo-science and the unintended consequences it creates among consumers who now fear perfectly safe and beneficial products."[24]

Hah. I've heard many outlandish things from Big Food companies, but I never thought I'd hear someone defend soda as "beneficial." It's also highly inappropriate for a company that peddles such an unhealthy product to lobby a government agency in such a manner.

Targeting Soda Critics. I'm not the first person to be targeted by Big Soda and I certainly won't be the last—they have a long history of going after their critics. Just look at what happened to Marion Nestle, a highly respected professor of nutrition at NYU and Cornell who wrote *Soda Politics*, a book about the devious marketing and lobbying efforts of Big Soda. As was made clear in a cache of e-mails published by Wikileaks, the Coca-Cola communication team was secretly tracking Professor Nestle's talks and lectures. They even snuck into her private events where she was talking with nutritionists. "Now I assume that someone from Coca-Cola is taking notes at every talk I give and reporting in to headquarters," Nestle says.[25]

One has to wonder: If the science is on their side, and soda really is safe and harmless, why is the soda industry so terrified of its critics?

ACTION STEPS: BREAK YOUR SODA HABIT

I hope you realize by now that Big Soda should not be trusted. If it were up to me, we'd make the soda aisle disappear. These drinks are not only a waste of money—they're making us sick. Being aware that you've been fed lies about soda is important. But it's even more important to just stop consuming this garbage.

Hopefully, I've convinced you that you'll feel better if you swear off all sodas, even those zero-calorie ones that pretend to be healthy. Before you can kick the habit, though, it's important to be honest about how many sodas you drink in a week. Add them up by keeping a food diary for seven days. For sticker shock, use a calculator to add up how many calories and sugar grams you're guzzling in that period. Take some time to think about the negative health consequences that you might suffer from drinking all that soda. Create a strong desire in your heart and mind to stop drinking soda and sweetened drinks—this is a very important step! If you really want to quit, you will succeed.

BUT DON'T TRY QUITTING ALL AT ONCE; EASE OFF SODA SLOWLY.

(These drinks have some addictive properties, especially when they're caffeinated.) Try cutting back by a fourth the first week, half the second week, and so on until you can quit soda completely. Each week you will be one step closer to meeting your goal and steadily improving your health.

Long-term success will ultimately depend on replacing soda with delicious alternatives. First, drink lots of clean, filtered water. (You'll be shocked at how much money you save by replacing soda with H_2O.) Purchase a refillable water bottle and keep it with you at home, at work, and in your car. Plus, find other fizz! Miss the refreshment and mouthfeel of sodas? Don't worry; you can still drink fizzy drinks that taste refreshing and are not loaded up with crappy chemicals. Just stay away from most store-bought versions and make your own drinks instead. Here are my favorite alternatives to soda:

- Organic raw kombucha
- Sparkling or soda water + lime juice + organic cranberry juice (with no added sugar or additives)
- Filtered water + fresh cucumbers + fresh or frozen strawberries
- Sparkling or soda water + fresh lemon or lime juice + grated ginger; consider adding melon, cucumbers, or berries for different flavors!
- 100 percent raw coconut water
- Organic unsweetened green and herbal tea (iced or hot); peppermint and ginger teas are great for satisfying cravings for something sweet

- Fresh pressed green juice; keep it low on the fruit, carrots, or beets

- Unsweetened coconut, cashew, or almond milk

- Coffee (iced or hot, with no sugar)

Avoiding soft drinks—even diet drinks—sends Big Soda a message that you're onto them. You know how to see through their lies. Instead of guzzling soda, you're going to stay hydrated with drinks that save you money and don't harm your vital organs.

What is sweeter than that?

CHAPTER 7:

"Free" Food: A High Cost to Health

My father has type 2 diabetes. The disease was caused, in part, by his love of fast food and candy. Growing up in India, he was raised to believe that food was scarce and that it should never, ever be wasted. As a result, he developed the habit of seeking out really cheap calories, which is why he ate so much McDonald's.

After he was diagnosed with diabetes, my father coped with the disease by seeking out "sugar-free" snacks that still satisfied his sweet tooth. I have many memories of walking with him into stores and watching him buy Glucerna shakes, a product marketed for diabetics as sugar free and as a suitable meal replacement. Because of the slick marketing, he also came under the spell of sugar-free snacks, such as Russell Stover sugar-free chocolates. They had no sugar, so they had to be safe, right? Isn't this what diabetics are supposed to eat?

My father learned about the dangers of these "sugar-free" foods the hard way. I'll never forget the call from my mother—I'd just learned I was pregnant and was giddy from happiness. But then my mother told me the terrible news: my father had been admitted to the hospital. The diabetes had begun affecting his brain. He couldn't think straight and lost control of his actions. These issues were caused by the fact that his blood sugar was wildly out of control, having clocked in at more than 300 for months. (Normal is around 98.)

How did this happen? At first, I was confused. Dad was just drinking sugar-free shakes and sugar-free treats. It didn't make sense that he'd have blood sugar issues.

But then I looked at the nutrition labels. Those Glucerna shakes might be sugar free, but they were chock full of man-made chemicals that had no business being marketed to ill people trying get well. Their very long ingredients list reads like a greatest hits of additives to avoid: there's tons of cellulose (which can disrupt our gut bacteria and cause inflammation), GMO soy fiber, GMO soy protein, fructose, GMO corn maltodextrin, and so on. It's a food made up entirely of chemicals you'd never eat on their own, or even find on a grocery store shelf.

Those sugar-free candies and desserts were no better. Even though he wasn't eating "sugar," after my dad visited his endo-crinologist it became clear that his "diabetic food" was nothing more than simple carbohydrates and sugar alcohols, which could also increase his blood sugar.[1] In short, the "sugar-free" foods were really dangerous, especially because they encourage people to consume way too many of them. The labels were selling a lie.

The good news is that after my dad stopped drinking these shakes and other processed diabetic food, his blood sugar sta-bilized and his brain started to function normally again. The dementia wasn't permanent; as the "sugar-free" foods cleared his system, he became himself again. I can't tell you how happy I was when I visited him in the hospital and he was calm, thoughtful, and clearheaded.

My father fell for the sugar free lie. But he's not the only one. At one time or another, we've all enjoyed some sugar-free ice cream, savored a few fat-free muffins, or told ourselves that those gluten-free cookies were healthier, so we could have one more. These choices seem like win-win foods: they taste like treats, but we don't have to deal with the guilt. If anything, we get to feel virtuous for having eaten so sensibly all day, right?

Not really. Most of these foods are actually loaded up with ingredients you definitely don't want in your body. I call this the "free" food fallacy: the labels make us think the foods are healthy, but they are anything but.

Their virtue is a lie.

WHY THE LIE?

The packaging on food has bamboozled us—and we're paying mightily for it by eating more calories and more junk than if we'd stuck to real, unprocessed food. In fact, studies show that when we nosh on these seemingly healthier alternatives, we tend to eat *twice* as much as we should. The end result is that Big Food makes a ton of money marketing cheap GMO ingredients as healthy while we're lining our arteries and other organs with harmful additives.

In order to understand why the "free" food fallacy is so dangerous, it's necessary to delve into the details. So let's examine the fallacy behind four major "free" labels and why "free" doesn't make a food healthy—and in fact, may do the opposite.

Test Your Food Label IQ

Do you ever buy products because of the flashy health claims on the label? Most of us are guilty of falling for claims on packages that say "natural" or "sugar free," believing that these products are superior to others on the shelf. I hate to say it, but you were probably conned. Take the following quiz to assess your label savvy and learn what labels really mean.

1. The term "no sugar added" means the same as "sugar free."
   - ❑ True
   - ❑ False

2. A food labeled "lightly sweetened" could have as many as 100 grams of sugar per serving.
   - ❏ True
   - ❏ False

3. A food labeled "all natural" may contain preservatives, genetically modified (GMO) ingredients, added sodium, or high-fructose corn syrup.
   - ❏ True
   - ❏ False

4. The term "multigrain" on a label means the food is healthier than foods labeled "whole grain" or "100% whole wheat."
   - ❏ True
   - ❏ False

5. A cereal "made with whole grains" is a healthy choice for obtaining the nutrients found in grains.
   - ❏ True
   - ❏ False

6. A food labeled "a good source of fiber" is as beneficial as the fiber found in whole grains and vegetables.
   - ❏ True
   - ❏ False

7. A food "made with real fruit" may have no whole fruit in it.
   - ❏ True
   - ❏ False

8. A product labeled cholesterol free also means the food is fat free.
   - ❏ True
   - ❏ False

9. A product can contain up to 0.5 grams of fat per serving and still be called "fat free."
   - ❏ True
   - ❏ False

10. Foods labeled "fat free" may contain as many (or more) calories as their full-fat counterparts.
    - ❏ True
    - ❏ False

Answers:

1. **False.** Here's the deal: this means exactly what the label says here, but it's easily misconstrued. "No sugar added" simply means they didn't add any sugar in the making of the product. That doesn't mean that it is sugar free, however, as it may still contain naturally occurring sugar. For instance, a "no sugar added" yogurt is still going to contain sugar in the form of lactose (which is a naturally occurring sugar in dairy).

   On the other hand, products with the "sugar free" label are typically heavily processed and are often sweetened with chemically derived artificial sweeteners or sugar alcohols. Be aware that they may contain up to 0.5 grams of sugars per serving, so they are not technically "free" of all sugar.

2. **True.** Not officially regulated by the FDA, this label indicates the food may contain 1 to 100 grams (maybe more) of sugar. For example, Starbucks Lightly Sweet Chai Tea Latte Grande has 31 grams of sugar!

3. **True.** "All natural" food doesn't mean what it should. The FDA hasn't formally defined how companies can use the natural label on their products, so that's why it is being exploited. At this point, the FDA considers a product "natural" when it doesn't contain any artificial colors, artificial flavors, or synthetic substances. However, a food labeled "natural" may still be chock full of GMOs, preservatives, and heavily processed ingredients like high-fructose corn syrup. The FDA is in the process of further defining this claim on packaging.

4. **False.** Whole grains (grains that are not refined, such as whole wheat, which contains the entire grain—the bran, the germ, and the endosperm) have more fiber and other nutrients than those that labeled multigrain. The "multigrain" label simply means multiple

different types of grains are used in the product, but these may be refined grains stripped of their nutrients and healthy fiber.

5. **False.** In reality, there might be only minute amounts of whole grains in these foods. They might also be made with refined corn flour (common in cereal), which spikes blood sugar a great deal and isn't at all good for you. To ensure you're getting the healthy, fiber-rich grains, check for "100% whole wheat" or "100% whole grains" on the label.

6. **False.** As this label is generally found on packaged foods, it indicates that the food contains a fiber additive. The industry calls these "functional fibers" but they do not function in your body the same as fiber found in real whole food because they don't contain the beneficial nutrients found in real whole food. We should be getting our fiber naturally from fruits, vegetables, beans, and seeds, and not from processed fiber additives that were manufactured in a lab.

7. **True.** Real fruit quantities aren't regulated by the FDA, so you could be buying a product with very little fruit in it. Some foods (like "fruit snacks") really just contain heavily processed fruit concentrates. To make a concentrate, the fruit is boiled down into a syrup, and this heating process destroys beneficial nutrients. When it comes to fruit, always try to eat the real thing!

8. **False.** The food may have no cholesterol, but it might be loaded with artery-clogging trans fats or other harmful fats.

9. **True.** A lot of people think "free" means it is completely "free" of something, but that's not always the case.

10. **True.** A muffin could be fat free, but might weigh in at 600 calories and be full of sugar. Most "fat free" foods are loaded with added sugar instead. Just because something is labeled "fat free," that doesn't give us the license to indulge.

THE TRUTH ABOUT "FREE" LABELS

The Sugar Free Label

Let's start with the "sugar free" label. Many sugar-free products are often just free of table sugar (sucrose) but may be laced with sugar alcohols or artificial sweeteners instead, including acesulfame potassium (Equal), saccharin (Sweet'N Low), aspartame (NutraSweet, Equal), and sucralose (Splenda). I discussed the health issues with these fake sweeteners in Chapter 5. They clearly should not be in our food and beverages.

Even more so, many sugar-free foods don't really save you calories, if that's your goal. Sugar-free brownies are a good example. A serving of regular Pillsbury chocolate brownies weighs in at 110 calories, while their "sugar-free" brownies have 90 calories. Not really much of a difference!

Sometimes chemically modified sugars are found in "sugar-free" foods. An example is maltodextrin, created from corn. (This is also found in those Pillsbury sugar-free brownies.) It's manipulated in a lab where it's broken down with enzymes to make it easier to digest. The easy digestibility of maltodextrin is where the problem lies. It digests as fast as pure sugar, which means that it can spike insulin levels in a similar way to sugar.[2]

Sugar-free foods often contain sugar alcohols. These additives can raise blood sugar levels too, just like they did in my father. Spiked blood sugar levels leads to *quickly* dropping blood sugar levels, which makes you crave even more carbs. It's a terrible hangover effect that leads many people to binge on these fake healthy snacks. In some people, sugar alcohols can also produce a laxative effect.

I'm convinced that one of the reasons the obesity epidemic is an especially critical issue in the United States is that we're hooked on these "sugar-free" foods. These products create an illusion of security that leads us to assume we can eat a lot of them without packing on pounds. We can't. They also train our taste buds to expect excessively sweet foods (I've found "sugar-free" treats sweetened with sugar alcohols taste *even sweeter* than their real sugar-sweetened counterparts), which creates a dangerous cycle of constant cravings. If you can't identify most of the ingredients on a food label, don't eat it.

Sugar might be toxic, but these alternatives are no better.

THE FAT FREE LABEL

If you don't eat fat, you can't get fat, right? Wrong. Foods that carry the "fat free" label trick you into believing that if you cut dietary fat out of your diet, your body fat will soon disappear too. Not true. The science shows that this rarely works.

The main reason is that when fat is removed from food, it is swapped out with carbohydrates (often refined sugar) or proteins processed in various ways with water or air to taste more like fat—all bad for the waistline!

Low-fat diets have been shown to be ineffective at producing lasting results. Even if dining on fat-free yogurt helps you shed a few pounds, the evidence shows that you're not really doing a body good. An extensive 2015 scientific review out of Harvard Medical School found that low-fat diets weren't any more effective than other types of diets that allow you to eat more fat.[3] Cutting fat grams simply doesn't coincide with less fat on your body. This is likely because low-fat and fat-free foods are typically full of refined sugar. Low-fat and fat-free yogurts, for instance, tend to be laden with more sugar than a scoop of ice cream.

That could explain why low-fat diets are also not necessarily good for the heart. Researchers in another large scientific review published in 2013 found that low-fat diets tend to increase triglycerides and decrease "good" (HDL) cholesterol in the body.[4] These two factors can put you at a bigger risk for heart disease. As was noted by Tufts researcher Dr. Dariush Mozaffarian in a 2016 issue of *Circulation*, "The lack of cardiometabolic benefit of low-fat diets has been convincingly demonstrated."[5]

Still, the failure of fat-free foods to make everybody skinny hasn't prevented the foods from invading every aisle of the grocery store, including some places they really shouldn't be.

Consider the "reduced fat" peanut butter made by Jif. Peanut butter should really be just 100 percent ground peanuts, but Jif claims their reduced-fat version is just 60 percent peanuts. What makes up the remaining 40 percent of the jar? Ingredients like corn syrup solids, sugar, pea protein, and fully hydrogenated oils. Yikes.

We shouldn't be afraid of the healthy fats in peanuts (and other natural foods like avocados, walnuts, and chia seeds). The Big Food industry has made us scared, supporting decades of misleading research, which has led people to seek out fat-free or low-in-fat foods. The end result is a dismal cycle: we buy these reduced-fat foods, which leave us less satisfied, which means we have to scarf down bigger servings and more sugar. It shouldn't be too surprising, then, that these "fat-free" foods make us even fatter.

THE TRANS FAT FREE LABEL

Now here's a type of fat that we should be avoiding, but it's not as easy as it seems. You may have heard in the news that the FDA finally banned "partially hydrogenated oils" from our food, a main source of trans fat. This is a step in the right direction— although a long time coming—because eating artificial trans fat is strongly correlated with an increased risk of type 2 diabetes and heart disease, and has been shown to lower good cholesterol and raise bad cholesterol levels.[6] The National Academy of Science's Institute of Medicine emphasizes that artificial trans fats have no known health benefit and there is no safe level to eat. *No safe level.*[7]

Partially hydrogenated oils should never have been allowed in our food in the first place. And it's not time for a celebration quite yet. The Big Food industry, it turns out, isn't quite ready to stop poisoning us with these cheap and deadly trans fats.

The reason is buried in the fine print. Although the FDA banned partially hydrogenated oils, they didn't address the other artificial additives in our food that also contain these heart-wrecking artificial trans fats. Some refined oils, emulsifiers, flavors, and colors contain trace amounts of trans fat, but they don't need to be labeled as such.

In fact, a very common emulsifier in processed food is one of these hidden sources of trans fat—and maybe you've heard of it: "mono- and diglycerides of fatty acids," or "monoglycerides" and "diglycerides." This additive helps keep oil and fat from separating, especially in processed foods. Unfortunately, these mono- and diglycerides are quickly converted by the body back into triglycerides, which are associated with heart disease. Even though mono- and diglycerides may contain trans fat, they aren't required to be labeled as trans fats on food packages because they are classified as emulsifiers, and can even be in food labeled "no trans fat."

The food industry has really exploited this loophole, adding mono- and diglycerides to a ton of foods that are labeled "no trans fat" and "0 grams of trans fat," such as Crisco shortening, and I Can't Believe It's Not Butter, light version. In fact, if you eat a lot of processed foods, monoglycerides and diglycerides are nearly impossible to avoid. This means that you are still eating trans fats even if you are taking pains to only eat trans fat–free foods.

You'll also have a hard time getting away from this ingredient if you're dining at mainstream and fast food restaurants, such as McDonald's, which uses the ingredient in its buns, shakes, ice cream, and biscuits. You also could be eating this ingredient at Burger King (croissants, specialty buns, frappes, and cookies) and Wendy's (Frosty and buns).

Why do most fast food restaurants use mono- and diglycerides? For the same reason processed food companies do: because it's cheap, it makes food last longer, and they can get away with it.

But it's time to stop the lie. When it comes to trans fats, even small amounts can be dangerous.

Flip It Over! When the Front of the Package Lies

I can't count how many times I've been shopping and found a product with a marketing claim on the front of the package that was so misleading that it was hardly true. Here are a few egregious examples:

Sargento Shredded Cheese—With the claim "Off the Block" blazoned on the front of the bag, they are insinuating this cheese is like the kind you'd shred "off the block" of cheese at home. Flipping it over to read the ingredients list, I found that it contains powdered cellulose, an additive made from wood and used as a coating on most pre-shredded cheese to keep it from sticking together. Eating cellulose is linked to weight gain, inflammation, and digestive problems. This is why I shred my own cheese!

Wishbone EVOO Salad Dressings—Right there in the product name you see that this dressing is full of healthy extra virgin olive oil, right? Well, not exactly. Right after olive oil, you'll find soybean oil listed on the ingredients list. This is closely followed by added sugar. Soybean oil is chemically refined, typically from GMO soybeans, and has an abundance of omega-6 fatty acids that increase the risk of inflammation, cardiovascular disease, cancer, and autoimmune diseases. So much for that healthy olive oil dressing!

RXBARs—The front of these healthy-looking bars lists their simple ingredients on the front: "3 egg whites, 6 almonds, 4 cashews, 2 dates, no B.S." What they don't tell you on the front, however, is that they also add natural flavors to their bars. You'll only find this disclosed when you read the real ingredients list on the back of the package. That sounds like a bit of B.S. to me. We'll learn in the next chapter why natural flavors don't belong in a real-food diet.

Canada Dry Ginger Ale—You'd think that ginger ale always contained ginger, right? Especially when the front of a bottle of Canada Dry Ginger Ale says it's "Made from Real Ginger." However, the ingredients list doesn't have ginger anywhere to be found. Instead, Canada Dry uses "natural flavors" that are derived from ginger. Why not just use actual ginger root and ditch the flavors?

> It's always important to flip products over to read the ingredients list and not make purchasing decisions based on the front of the package. That's where you'll find the real truth.

THE GLUTEN FREE LIE

Strolling the supermarket, I see shelves groaning with products proclaiming their freedom from gluten: bread, pasta, crackers, cookies, cereal, beer, and others. Gluten free is what low carb was years ago: The "in" diet discussed on talk shows and bestsellers, promoted by high-profile celebs, and followed by the masses. "Gluten free" is part of the new dieting vocabulary, and it's all the rage.

But unlike other dietary demons such as bad carbs or bad fat, gluten is not inherently harmful for everyone. Only a small percentage of the population can't properly digest this protein, which occurs naturally in wheat, barley, and rye and is a natural substance that gives certain foods their structure.

The hype around gluten free has generated a lot of misinformation, including a couple of big lies. One is that eliminating gluten from your diet will help you lose weight. Another is that going gluten free is healthier.

Neither of these claims has been proven. But this hasn't slowed the growth of gluten-free products. Gluten-free product sales have increased dramatically in recent years, raking in billions of dollars.

While gluten-free eating has been a bit trendy in recent years, for some people it is a medical requirement. Gluten affects some people adversely, notably those with celiac disease, an autoimmune disorder that afflicts approximately 1 percent of the population.[8] With this disease, the body treats gluten as a poison. When gluten is eaten, a person with celiac will experience abnormal inflammation in the body, leading to intestinal damage. If left untreated, this may lead to malnutrition, as the body is not able to properly absorb nutrients from food.

Diagnosing celiac disease or a gluten or wheat intolerance should be performed by a knowledgeable physician. According to the Celiac Disease Foundation, a simple blood test is available to screen for celiac disease. It identifies certain antibodies in the blood. These antibodies are produced by the immune system because it views gluten (the proteins found in wheat, rye, and barley) as a threat.[9]

"Anyone who suffers from an unexplained, stubborn illness for several months, should consider celiac disease a possible cause and be properly screened for it," advises the Celiac Disease Center at Columbia University Medical Center.[10]

Some people have less severe gluten allergies or sensitivities—maybe 7 or 8 percent of the U.S. population. Even so, about 30 percent of adults in the U.S. are either trying to avoid gluten, or ease back on it, says the marketing firm NPD Group.[11] That means a lot of people avoiding gluten-free foods really don't need to. This wouldn't be a problem except that many whole foods containing gluten are packed with nutritional benefits. And many gluten-free foods are full of processed junk.

There are three common pitfalls of a gluten-free diet, unless you have celiac disease or a diagnosed intolerance to gluten:

Gluten free doesn't mean guilt free. There's simply no proof that eliminating gluten from your diet will help you lose weight. When people with celiac disease start a gluten-free diet, their digestion greatly improves over time and it's common for them to gain some weight. This is healthy for them, and means they are healing.

When someone without celiac loses weight after ditching gluten, it's likely because they stopped eating all those processed foods they used to eat (refined breads, pastas, crackers) that happen to be loaded with gluten, but that doesn't make gluten the culprit. If you get a little thinner on a gluten-free diet, it's most likely because you're cutting back on many fattening and processed high-calorie foods such as fried foods, pizza, crackers, and breads. This is a good thing. But it's not the gluten that's holding you back—it's the processed foods.

Speaking of calories, many gluten-free products can be higher in calories than gluten-containing foods. This occurs when food manufacturers replace the missing gluten with extra fat and sugar.

Gluten free can have extra additives. The gluten-free fad has given rise to an entire industry of gluten-free convenience foods that contain questionable additives and preservatives, refined sugar, and nutrient-empty ingredients. For instance, in gluten-free products you might find yourself eating:

Tapioca Starch. One of the main ingredients used to replace wheat flour. It is very high in carbohydrates but hardly contains any fiber, fat, protein, vitamins, or minerals, and basically just supplies empty calories that can spike blood sugar higher and faster than refined sugar.

Rice Starch, Rice Flour, and Brown Rice Syrup. Rice is very common in gluten-free diets, but it's notoriously contaminated with arsenic, which is a poison and a potent human carcinogen. Arsenic is also classified as a group 1 carcinogen by the International Agency for Research on Cancer.[12]

In 2012, *Consumer Reports* tested more than 200 products and found significant levels of arsenic in several brands of rice (especially brown), rice pasta, rice flours, rice cereals, rice crackers, brown rice syrup, and rice cakes. This can be a problem in gluten-free diets because rice is found in so many gluten-free foods.[13]

Corn and Soy. Corn and soy ingredients (corn meal, corn starch, corn syrup, soybean oil, and soy lecithin) are found in a lot of gluten-free pastas, crackers, and cookies. When you see anything made from conventional corn or soy on a label, it's a pretty safe bet that it's genetically modified because the vast majority of these crops in the U.S. are GMO. Roundup-ready GMO crops are sprayed with the herbicide glyphosate, which has been shown to accumulate in the crops. This is scary because glyphosate has been deemed a "probable carcinogen" by the World Health Organization.[14] It is also believed to destroy healthy gut bacteria.[15] I definitely don't want it sprayed on my food. Do you?

Added Sugar. Gluten-free foods use sugar to replace the flavors lost when grains are removed. It's virtually impossible to find a gluten-free product without added refined sugar. In fact, you'll often see sugar listed several times on the "gluten-free" ingredients list in its many different forms: corn syrup, maltodextrin, dextrin, sugar, and so forth. Also, beware that unless the ingredient label says "cane sugar," it is likely sugar from GMO sugar beets.

Xanthan Gum. When the gluten is removed from baked goods, food companies often add the additive xanthan gum for texture and softness. This hasn't really been shown to be a dangerous ingredient to consume, but be aware that it's often derived from GMO corn and triggers allergies or gastrointestinal issues in susceptible people. If I see this on an ingredients list, it may not be a deal breaker, but I try my best to avoid it and seek out the non-GMO variety.

Gluten free can lead to deficiencies. Gluten-free foods are not necessarily healthier or better for you (unless you have celiac disease or a true gluten intolerance). A 2015 study published in the *British Journal of Nutrition* evaluated the nutritional value of gluten-free and non–gluten free foods in core food groups. Researchers evaluated a total of 3,213 food products, and foods rated on a scale from low nutritional value to high nutritional value. The researchers found that gluten-free foods were lower in nutrients, concluding that: "The consumption of gluten-free products is unlikely to confer health benefits, unless there is clear evidence of gluten intolerance."[16]

Another study published in the *Journal of the American Dietetic Association* found that people on strict gluten-free diets were not eating enough fiber, iron, or calcium.[17] By eating gluten-free foods when you don't need to, you can become deficient in several nutrients. In contrast, whole-grain foods have many health benefits. Notably, they're rich in B vitamins and iron. Whole grains are also excellent sources of dietary fiber, which is imperative for good digestion and gut health. This means that if you need to remove gluten from your diet, you have to be diligent in finding other sources for these healthful nutrients.

ACTION STEPS: GO GLUTEN FREE THE RIGHT WAY

If you have celiac or feel better on a gluten-free diet, what's the best way to ensure it's as healthy as possible? You probably already know what I'm about to say, but here's the kick in the pants that you may need: don't buy processed gluten-free replacement foods that can sabotage your health. Instead of buying gluten-free breads and crackers filled with additives and sugar, fill your diet with healthy whole foods that are *naturally* gluten free (vegetables, fruits, beans, seeds, lentils, nuts) to nourish your body. These foods constitute a very healthy way to eat, something that has been known for decades.

Because going gluten free is very important for many people, here are my recommendations:

- Get to know ancient grains. Cultivated for thousands of years, ancient grains represent some of the oldest grains consumed by humans. They include quinoa, amaranth, millet, teff, and sorghum. Many are gluten free and packed with vitamins, minerals, fiber, and protein. These delicious grains also offer tremendous benefits, such as preventing cancer, heart disease, and high blood pressure.

- Instead of using a gluten-free tortilla, make a wrap out of collard greens. The individual leaves can be blanched to take on the texture of a tortilla, and they are so much healthier.

- Choose pastas that are made from lentils or beans, like those from Tolerant Pasta, or make your own "noodles" out of spaghetti squash, or zucchini using a spiralizer.

- Substitute quinoa for rice when making stir-fries and other dishes that are typically served over rice. This will help minimize your exposure to arsenic.

- Use baking recipes that primarily call for flours with healthy nutrients such as coconut flour, almond meal, buckwheat flour, quinoa flour, chickpea flour, teff flour, or sorghum flour. Sometimes these are mixed with a bit of tapioca flour for texture; just make sure you are using nutritious flours as well.

- If you can't bake your own bread, seek out store-bought breads that are made primarily from nutrient-rich ancient grains or buckwheat (and rely less on rice or tapioca flours).

- Make your pizza crusts from cauliflower. Sounds crazy, right? But cauliflower blends up with goat cheese and eggs into a great dough for pizza that's packed with nutrients. Cauliflower also can be blended up in a food processor into "rice" that you just sauté for a few minutes to make the perfect rice substitute.

- For snacks, choose bars that are made with organic seeds, nuts, and dried fruit.

- Last but not least: eat more produce! Fruit, veggies, beans, and salad greens are all naturally gluten free, so don't be afraid to try new ones every week until you find your favorites.

The gluten-free craze will soon fade, just like every diet fad before it. But I hope what lasts is the larger trend toward eating natural, whole foods such as vegetables, fruits, nuts, seeds, legumes, and sources of lean protein. This natural diet might not have a lot of marketing muscle behind it—when was the last time you saw a billboard for broccoli?—but it will keep you healthy and energetic for a lifetime.

Other "Freebies"	
Label	**What It Really Means**
Dairy Free	This term does not have a regulatory definition. The Food Allergy Research & Resource Program has found products labeled "dairy free" that contain milk. These products may also contain milk derivatives (such as whey).
Nondairy	The label "nondairy" has a regulatory definition; however, it expressly allows for milk protein to be used in products. For example, you may find a "nondairy" coffee creamer that doesn't contain cream but still contains caseinate (a milk derivative).
Lactose Free	This label means that lactose, a milk sugar, has been removed, but the rest of the milk could still be there. If you're a vegan or a dairy-free person, lactose free is still not for you, since these products are still milk based.
Sodium Free, and Other Sodium Labels	There are various labels describing the presence of salt in foods: sodium free means there is a very small amount of sodium per serving (less than 5 mg); very low sodium (35 mg or less per serving); low sodium (140 mg or less per serving); reduced sodium (the level of sodium is reduced by 25%); light in sodium (sodium is reduced by at least 50%); and no salt is added (no salt added during processing, but can still contain sodium from other sources). The easiest way to determine the sodium load of a food is to check the Nutrition Facts label for how many grams it contains per serving.
Grain Free	Grain free means the product contains no ingredients that are grains, such as wheat, rice, corn, barley, and oats. However, that does not mean the product is gluten free because it could still contain gluten from processing contamination or additives.
Wheat Free	Wheat free does not mean the same as gluten free; they have very different meanings. Wheat free means there are no wheat ingredients (such as whole-wheat or all-purpose flour) in a food, but it could still contain other ingredients that contain gluten.

ACTION STEPS: READ PAST THE HYPE ON FOOD PACKAGING

Don't be fooled by "free" labels. They reflect a lot of hype and say nothing about the nutritional quality of the food. A 2017 study in the *Journal of the Academy of Nutrition and Dietetics* examined the nutrient claims on over 80 million food and beverage purchases in the U.S. between 2008 and 2012.[18] The researchers found that 13 percent of food and 35 percent of beverages purchased had some sort of "low content claim" on the package. Low fat, low calorie, and low sugar were the most common claims found on packages. That being said, consumers were not getting exactly what they thought they paid for. Many of these products were found to have an inferior nutritional profile compared to products that don't make such claims. The researchers concluded that low content–labeled foods "may mislead about the overall nutritional quality of the food." So "free" foods can be the least nutritious foods to choose.

I read food labels closely. It's the best way to know what's truly in a packaged food and whether it's good for you. Reading food ingredients lists carefully may take time and prolong your trips to the grocery store, but if you care about your health, it's well worth the time and effort. Plus, practice makes perfect; the more you do it, the faster you'll get. Once you learn how to see through the lies, you can see the truth pretty quickly.

A lot of people think you shouldn't blame food companies or anyone else for these lies. After all, they're just trying to sell their products! What's wrong with a little marketing?

But I think many of these "free" food fallacies go well beyond marketing. They are targeting people most in need of eating healthy food. People like my father. When companies practice this type of label trickery, when they cram fake sugars into "sugar-free" foods, and way too much real sugar into "fat-free" foods, and trans fats additives into "trans fat–free" foods, and all sorts of junk into "gluten-free" foods, it becomes clear that they don't care about our health. All they care about is their profits.

So you have a choice. You can let the food companies dupe you. You can keep on paying for junk foods wrapped in deceptive packaging. Or you can treat them like the enemy and stop buying their products. Vote with your dollars—not just once in a while but *always*. Your health is the only thing you've got.

I'm thankful it wasn't too late for my father; he was able to stop drinking those sugar-free shakes and recover his mind. He gets to play with his granddaughter. But for too many Americans, these food lies are doing irreparable harm.

CHAPTER 8

Flavor:
It's Not Natural

The news that RXBARs decided to place their ingredients label on the front of their packaging stunned me as if I had walked into a glass door. A few years ago, I predicted that companies would make this move because consumers care about ingredients. I shared my prediction with the ex-CEO of Whole Foods after he asked me about future trends in food packaging.

At first, I was delighted at the thought my prediction had come true. But upon closer inspection of the RXBAR labels (even the ones for kids), I was shattered. While the packaging has the appearance of transparency—the company brags that "one look at our wrapper, and you can see what we're all about"—I noticed that the back of the label had its own ingredients list in small print, which included "natural flavors," a term that not only raises my eyebrows but keeps them up there all night. Why doesn't RXBARs list "natural flavors" on the front of their package like the other ingredients? My guess is that it's because they know the truth about this suspicious ingredient and don't want to put a spotlight on it.

In a subsequent e-mail from the company, they told me, "Natural flavors are purified extracts from natural sources, such as a spice, fruit, or vegetables. In order to be used in food, natural flavors must meet strict FDA guidelines and safety criteria. The natural flavors used in RXBARs come from the real food ingredients such as fruit and chocolate and do not include propylene glycol, synthetic, artificial or GMO derived ingredients." While this is helpful information, it does not excuse the fact that they don't list "natural flavors" on the front of the package along with the other ingredients. I find this highly misleading. We also still don't really know what's in those flavors. Why can't RXBARs use just 100 percent real food? This was around the time I started to question what even the health food industry was doing to my food and began considering taking matters into my own hands.

In the fall of 2017, I started Truvani, my own food product line. It was a move I'd been resisting for years. Although I'd been approached countless times by executives in the food industry eager to brand foods with the Food Babe label, I'd always said no. And that's because I saw myself as an outsider. I was an advocate for healthy foods. I was worried that if I became part of the food industry, I would lose the ability to fight for better products.

At a certain point, however, I realized that it wasn't enough to fight from the outside. My epiphany began with yogurt. For a while, I'd been enjoying a grass-fed vanilla yogurt from an organic dairy farm. But then the small company got bought by a bigger manufacturer. They promised to maintain their principles but then, a few months later, I noticed that the yogurt now contained a bunch of thickening additives, and they had replaced real vanilla with "natural flavors."

This same story has played out so many times over the years. A company starts out with great intentions. The company gets acquired. Then, the company changes their ingredients to cut costs. It's frustrating. It makes me really angry and sad. Isn't our health worth a few extra pennies?

And that's when I decided that this would happen for the last time. Although being an activist had produced real change, it still hadn't led to products that I wanted to consume. We'd gotten rid of plenty of bad stuff, but too many products were still missing the good stuff.

So I finally came to the conclusion that I needed to create what I wanted to eat. The mission of our new food company would be simple: we would sell real food without added chemicals, products without toxins, and labels without lies. This would be food I'd be proud to feed my family.

The process has been very educational, to say the least! The first thing I learned was just how hard it is to source real, healthy ingredients. While I knew it might be a bit more expensive to get the good stuff, I couldn't believe the price difference. It was also much more difficult to source clean ingredients that passed our rigorous tests for toxins, pesticides, and heavy metals.

And that's when I truly began to understand the shortcuts taken by nearly every food product you find in the grocery store. These Big Food companies don't fight for the best ingredients, which is why it is so hard for us to find good suppliers. And they certainly don't spend the extra money on sourcing foods that are healthy and delicious.

Why not?

Because they don't need to. These companies know they can get away with selling us cheap junk because of a dirty secret: *the flavor industry.*

We are being targeted.

I bet if you go to your kitchen cabinet right now and pick up the first food package you see, you'll find the word "flavor" somewhere on the ingredients list. Am I right?

Yep, the processed food industry adds flavors to almost everything. Wonder why? When a food is heavily processed with machinery in a factory, pumped full of preservatives, and poured into a package that gets shipped across the country to get stored on a shelf for months, it loses flavor. That's why there is a multibillion-dollar flavor industry dedicated to creating chemicals that make all that processed food taste like . . . well . . . real food.

Not only do these flavors make fake food taste real, but they also give it a special "kick." The natural and artificial chemicals that flavor manufactures engineer have been synthesized to trick your mind into wanting more and more. Why do Americans eat more calories than any other industrialized nation? It's not because we have more money or are more hungry. It's because our food supply is chemically produced and enhanced with these "flavors" and they're *everywhere*—and we are being *targeted*.

You see, they don't want you to have the full essence of the strawberry; they want you to only experience the best 1 millionth part of the taste, so you get "addicted" and keep having to go back for more and more, searching continuously for gratification—eating more of that product, which in turns fills Big Food's pockets. Big Food is hijacking your taste buds one by one.

FLAVOR: IT'S FAR FROM NATURAL

The notion that the added flavors in our food are natural is a lie. The term "flavors" on a package is highly misleading. It sounds innocent and is on so many products that we are desensitized to it. Flavor companies own these proprietary formulas, making it nearly impossible to find out exactly what's in them.

You'd like to think that "natural apple flavor" is just some juice extracted from an apple and inserted into the food. Nope. That "natural apple flavor" needs to be preserved and stabilized and has agents added to help it mix well into a product. This is why flavors can contain upward of 100 different chemicals, like propylene glycol, polysorbate 80, BHT, BHA . . . all considered "incidental additives" not required to be labeled by the FDA.[1] The FDA doesn't require companies to tell you what is in the flavors they use. It's a complete mystery ingredient. I'd like to know if my vanilla yogurt secretly contained butylated hydroxyanisole (a preservative banned in foreign countries and linked to cancer[2]), wouldn't you? In natural flavors, their secret is safe. It's quite the racket.

Hint flavored water was hit with a lawsuit because their drinks—which boast they only contain "natural flavors from non-GMO plants"—tested positive for propylene glycol, an artificial solvent frequently used by the flavoring industry. Wouldn't you rather just drink plain water with a squeeze of lemon? It's not only much cheaper—I'd argue it's much better for you.

Natural flavor can also legally contain naturally occurring "glutamate," an additive that mimics MSG, a known excitotoxin. Excitotoxins can have far-reaching and damaging effects on the body. They infiltrate the bloodstream and can overexcite cells throughout the nervous system. Worst of all, excitotoxins also make food irresistible to eat and can thus contribute to obesity.

Then there are the "yuck factor" natural flavorings, such as castoreum, a substance used to augment some strawberry and vanilla flavorings. It comes from "rendered beaver anal gland." (What, you don't want beaver butt with your strawberry protein bar?)

So-called "natural" flavorings can also be laced with GMO-derived ingredients (unless the food is organic or Non-GMO Project verified).

There is absolutely no health benefit provided by these natural flavors; they are not adding any extra nutritional value to your food. Most of the time, they are simply there to cover up the highly processed nature of what you're eating.

Taken together, these facts are proof that natural flavors are not natural, and they're definitely not good for you.

Who Is Overseeing the Safety of Flavors in Our Food? You May Be Surprised . . .

The fox is guarding the henhouse. You see, there is no governmental or independent agency that approves or oversees the safety of the food flavors. Instead, a flavor industry trade group, the Flavor and Extract Manufacturers Association (FEMA), has assembled their own panel of scientists who review and approve new flavors as Generally Recognized as Safe (GRAS). These scientists are paid by FEMA (who ultimately get their funding from flavor companies).[3]

And, of course, the FEMA panel scientists are supposed to be independent and free of conflicts of interest, but many questions have been raised about their closed-door evaluations and lack of transparency with the public. The fact that this panel is assembled and paid for by a flavor company trade group is concerning to say the least, don't you think?

Public advocacy groups have questioned FEMA's processes and called on the FDA to ban certain flavor substances that have known links to cancer,[4] but little has been done. Some chemicals used to make flavors, like diacetyl (which is used to make buttery flavor), are highly dangerous for those that work around them . . . but we are supposed to eat them and be okay? Consumers want to know what's in these flavors and what research has been done proving their safety, but we essentially get the door slammed in our faces when we ask. This is yet another reason to be wary of the flavors in your food.

WHY THE LIE?

Food companies know they can get us hooked on junk food—and one of the ways they do it is by creating tantalizing food flavors in food labs and then lying to us about how natural those flavors are. They know that consumers prefer "natural" because "artificial" has the wrong connotations and doesn't sell.

Because of flavor technology, processed food can be addictive. I confess that once in a while, I crave Annie's Chocolate Bunnies. Once I open the box, I literally can't stop eating them. (I'm thinking about them right now, and my mouth is watering.) It's like these little cookies short-circuit my self-control.

But here's the strange twist: I don't have the same gotta-have-it feeling when I make homemade cookies. Although my homemade cookies are delicious, I don't want to eat the whole batch at once. It's only those chocolate bunnies that I can't resist.

What's going on? Why can't I stop? Is it the sugar?

Turns out, it's way more than just sugar. Not long ago, I sat down with Mark Schatzker, author of the acclaimed book *The*

Dorito Effect.[5] The book borrows its title from the tortilla chip that became a nationwide sensation after it was flavored with a delectable taco taste. In his book, Schatzker delves into the reasons why food doesn't taste the way it used to. The story begins with the move toward mass production, which requires Big Food to skimp on quality ingredients for the sake of higher profits. Instead of seeking out deliciousness, Big Food focuses on yield, pest resistance, and cost. It doesn't matter if you're looking at tomatoes, strawberries, wheat, or broccoli: the food industry has systematically bred out flavor in pursuit of more practical "virtues," like whether or not a tomato can be shipped thousands of miles without bruising.

There are two big problems with this approach. First, it makes our food less nutritious. When we breed crops to satisfy the Big Food industry, we end up growing fruits and vegetables with dramatically fewer health benefits.

The second problem is that those industrial ingredients lead to really bland food. (There's nothing tasty about GMO corn and soy by-products. And those mass-grown tomatoes usually taste like cardboard.) To compensate for this blandness, Big Food companies have engineered ways to make synthetic flavors that are so enticing and addictive we can't stop eating them.

Take Doritos. They started out as a plain tortilla chip with a little salt, hardly like the ones you'll find in stores today. This inaugural version of the chip was a market failure; sales were dismal because they didn't taste like much. However, a marketing executive at Frito-Lay named Arch West decided that the chips would sell better if they were coated in an intense orange powder that resembles taco flavor.[6] And thus was the modern Dorito born, a food that has become a template for countless other highly processed junk food products that hide their tasteless ingredients by dousing them with tasty chemicals.

These chemical flavors can save the companies a huge amount of money. I was recently in a supermarket and came across some blueberry English muffins. Sounds fairly healthy, right? But here's the catch: the muffins contained no actual blueberries. Instead, the ingredients listed something called "blueberry flavored bits," which were made of sugar, wheat flour, natural and artificial flavors, Blue #2, and Red #40. Sugar and blue dye, I guess, are cheaper than real berries.

And it's not just blueberries. Dannon Oikos Triple Zero strawberry yogurt contains zero strawberries. (They trick you into thinking otherwise by adding some vegetable juice concentrate for red color and "natural flavors.") Although they position the yogurt as a healthy food with "0 fat" and "no added sugar," wouldn't it be healthier to eat some real berries with your yogurt?

Or consider vanilla. If you see vanilla flavor in a mass-produced product, chances are it's just a "natural flavor" and not the real thing. Why? Because the real thing is expensive: a pound of pure vanillin (from vanilla beans) costs $1,200. Big Food, however, can create that same flavor for about $6 a pound, which is why so many products, from those yogurts to baked goods, rely instead on this fake flavor.

Diet Coke recently came out with four enticing new flavors: Zesty Blood Orange, Feisty Cherry, Twisted Mango, and Ginger Lime, which are designed to appeal to a younger generation. But you'll find no actual blood orange, cherry, mango, ginger, or lime in these drinks. In fact, they all have a nearly identical ingredients list to original Diet Coke (complete with caramel color, aspartame, and phosphoric acid), each spiked with a new "natural flavor." They've simply taken an old product and repackaged it as something new and trendy.

This is the Dorito model of modern food and it's been a catastrophe for our health. By making junk food palatable, the flavor industry has helped drive the obesity epidemic, not to mention high rates of heart disease and type 2 diabetes.

Because the famous Frito-Lay slogan "Betcha can't eat just one" is essentially true: these counter-nutritional snacks are expressly designed to make you want to eat the whole bag. In an interview with *60 Minutes*,[7] flavor scientists from Givaudan, one of the leading flavor companies in the world, essentially admitted that one of their chief goals was making food addictive:

Givaudan scientist #1: In our fruit flavors we're talking about, we want a burst in the beginning. And maybe a finish that doesn't linger too much so that you want more of it.

Givaudan scientist #2: And you don't want a long linger, because you're not going to eat more of it if it lingers.

60 Minutes **reporter:** Aha. So I see, it's going to be a quick fix. And then—

Givaudan scientist #1: Have more.

60 Minutes **reporter:** And then have more. But that suggests something else?

Givaudan scientist #1: Exactly.

60 Minutes **reporter:** Which is called addiction?

Givaudan scientist #1: Exactly.

60 Minutes **reporter:** You're tryin' to create an addictive taste?

Givaudan scientist #1: That's a good word.[8]

You want salad dressing on your salad? You want a little mustard or mayo on your sandwich? Some salsa with your chips? These products are all laced with "natural flavors," designed to keep us stuffing our face with food that would otherwise be bland and boring. But I don't want to eat foods that trick my taste buds into downing almost a whole box in one sitting (like those Annie's Bunnies!) or make real food seem like second best. I like to know exactly what I'm eating, and with "natural flavors" I'm left in the dark. Sticking with real food is just simpler, healthier, and oftentimes cheaper too.

Flavor Cheat Sheet

There are some stark differences between artificial flavors, natural flavors, natural strawberry flavors, organic raspberry flavors, and others. And while these are all largely the same, some of the flavors added to food are better than others. Here's a summary of what these mean when you see them on a label. (Note: "X" stands for a specific flavor, such as "strawberry" or "vanilla.")

Artificial Flavors or Artificial "X" Flavors	Artificial flavors are chemical mixtures made with synthetic (not natural) ingredients in a lab. They're produced by fractional distillation and chemical manipulation of various chemicals like crude oil or coal tar. Artificial vanilla flavor can be made from wood pulp. With artificial flavors, chemists can make anything taste like a strawberry without any actual strawberries (or any actual food, for that matter), which is a really horrible thing if you care about health. But it's a great thing for food manufacturers because artificial flavors are much cheaper than using real food (or even natural flavors).
Natural Flavors	Natural flavor is practically the exact same thing as artificial flavor, but it's derived from substances found in nature (plants, animals, etc.). So, the flavor is derived from natural things, but it's important to remember that this isn't all it contains. Remember: flavors typically contain preservatives, emulsifiers, solvents, and other "incidental additives" that can make up 80% or so of the formulation, even the "natural" ones. Flavor chemists create these complex formulations in a lab, isolating and blending specific flavors extracted from upward of hundreds of compounds, some of which may be GMOs. These compounds can come from substances that are nowhere close to the actual thing. For example, they might take some castoreum from a beaver to make a flavoring that resembles a raspberry—without ever using any raspberries. But, hey, it's "natural" because it's from a beaver.

Natural "X" Flavor	In general, if you see something like "natural cinnamon flavor," this means that the flavor is derived solely from the named fruit, vegetable, animal, or plant, which in this case is cinnamon. In other words, if you see "natural raspberry flavor" on a product, the flavor didn't come from a beaver, but actual raspberries. Incidental additives still apply, of course.
Natural and Artificial "X" Flavor*	You'll see a label like this when there are both natural and artificial flavors in a product. It doesn't necessarily mean any of the named source (i.e., a cherry) is used.
"X" Flavor, with Other Natural Flavor	Sometimes on the front of a package you'll see the statement "raspberry flavor with other natural flavor" . . . which sounds redundant. This means the food contains a flavor derived from raspberries, but also other natural flavors that don't come from raspberries. This doesn't need to be disclosed on an ingredients list but is required on the front panel of the package if they want to describe the flavor on the front.
Organic Natural Flavor	A lot of people are surprised that organic foods can contain natural flavors. While it's not ideal, at least "organic natural flavor" is made just like other organic ingredients and needs to follow the same regulations. That means that organic flavors won't contain synthetic solvents or preservatives. Some of the "incidental additives" banned from organic flavors include propylene glycol, mono- and diglycerides, BHT, BHA, and polysorbate 80.
Natural Flavors (in a "USDA Certified Organic" Product)	Sometimes you'll just see "natural flavors" listed on a Certified Organic product (instead of "Organic Natural Flavors"). This means that the flavor itself is not organic, but it is compliant with organic regulations, such as no synthetic ingredients or GMOs. So, ultimately, these flavors will have a cleaner profile than the average natural flavor.

NATURAL FLAVORS = NO NUTRITION

I highlighted my copy of *The Dorito Effect* like crazy and immediately reached out to Schatzker because I was so impressed with the investigative work he has done. Here are some of the takeaways from our conversation:[9]

True natural flavor is an indicator of nutrition to animals—and was also to us, apparently, before our palates were tricked and befuddled by junk food. Both animals and human infants demonstrate considerable "nutritional wisdom" when left to their own devices. Schatzker described a riveting 1926 experiment that allowed children to select their own foods for six years. While you might think the kids binged on sweet stuff, they all ended up settling on extremely nutritious and balanced diets. One girl had liver and orange juice for breakfast; a boy with rickets would guzzle cod liver oil occasionally until he got over the illness. In the end, the children in this group were markedly healthier than those fed by nutritionists.

That's because flavor in nature is almost always a mark of nutrition. Flavors are the cue that tells us where to find the nutrients we need. For example, the flavors we love in tomatoes are synthesized from essential nutrients like beta carotene, amino acids, and omega-3s. The flavor, in other words, is a chemical sign that tells your brain there's good stuff in here—you should eat one.

Junk food turns this healthy instinct against us. Our stores are full of foods that taste like all kinds of different things but don't come with the same nutrients. You can create a food that tastes like a tomato or blueberry without any nutritional value at all—and that's a problem.

Those natural flavors can also make you eat things you wouldn't normally eat. Soda without flavors is just carbonated water and sugar. No one would drink that without the flavors added. It's not just the sugar; flavor is the missing piece of the puzzle.

In recent years, "flavor chemistry" has become a huge business and highly specialized science. Schatzker, for example, explains how Big Food can engineer the flavor of a blueberry without using any actual blueberries. They begin by identifying the key chemical compounds that give rise to that wonderful blueberry flavor. Of course, real blueberries are expensive, so the companies don't want to get those compounds from the healthy fruit. Instead, they seek out cheaper sources for these same compounds, such as tree bark, grass, and yeast. "When the process is complete, you have a test tube full of pure chemicals, none of which came from an actual blueberry," Schatzker writes. "Chemically speaking, these compounds are identical to an artificial blueberry flavoring. But the government says you can label it natural."[10] That's how we end up with "blueberry flavored bits" in English muffins that are made up of sugar, flavoring, and artificial dyes, with absolutely no blueberries.

I must emphasize that natural flavors aren't necessarily toxic. I think the biggest hazard added flavors pose, by far, is the way they create food addictions and entice us to eat junk. What they do is tantalize us to eat unhealthy foods in unhealthy quantities. We all think we have the mental ability to control what we eat, but flavor technology makes us crave foods we wouldn't normally go near. Eating these foods in excess (like unhealthy soda or chips) can make you sick and maybe send you to an early grave.

Don't be fooled. "Natural flavors" may sound harmless but that doesn't mean they're good for you.

The Dangers of a Whiff of Flavor: Popcorn Workers' Lungs

Food companies might not want to publicize all the details about "flavors," but some emit toxic fumes, putting flavor company employees in harm's way. In particular, the flavoring ingredient diacetyl has been linked to lung disease among employees at flavoring production facilities.[11] This chemical was commonly used to give a fake buttery flavor to microwave popcorn; thus the medical condition it caused was coined "popcorn lung." It's rare and irreversible, and there's no good treatment for the disease short of a lung transplant. Since this was discovered, major food manufacturers have eliminated this chemical from their flavors.

We don't know what these manufacturers have substituted for diacetyl, and there's the possibility that some brands still use it because it hasn't been banned. A possible substitute for diacetyl is 2,3-pentanedione, which is also linked to lung damage in animal studies.

2,3-pentanedione and diacetyl are designated "generally recognized as safe" by the FDA for use in foods. But here are my questions: If these flavor chemicals are too dangerous to inhale, why would we want to swallow them? And why are food companies willing to put the health of their workers at risk to save a buck? Flavors might be cheap, but are they worth the cost of worker health?

ACTION STEPS: FIGHT FLAVORING

The food industry's flavor trickery makes it really important (and hard) to be a smart consumer. When looking at your food, ask yourself, as Mark Schatzker expertly says, "Did *someone* engineer this to be delicious or did *nature* engineer this to be delicious?"

Remember that the word "natural" on a product is virtually bogus. It doesn't equate with good. Take time to read the ingredients list found on the package, and read the fine print. If they list artificial or natural flavors, put those foods back on the shelf and look for an alternative. Feel free to call up a company and ask questions. Look for products that use real food to flavor their products. Above all, let's stop food companies and flavor factories from getting us hooked on processed foods.

As for me, I've learned to stop buying Annie's Chocolate Bunnies. I don't know why I can't resist them. But one look at the ingredients list with "natural flavor" tells me that I probably should.

I'm going to bake some homemade cookies instead.

CHAPTER 9

Fortified
Food Fraud

Big Food has been remarkably effective at convincing people that certain processed foods are good for us. The list of such foods is long: instant breakfast shakes, sports drinks, fiber bars, and countless other processed food products are marketed using the language of health and well-being. Oftentimes, people are eating toxic crap but are convinced these foods will make them feel better, perform better, and avoid illness.

Perhaps the best example of this con—tricking people into thinking junk food is good for us—has been the invention of breakfast cereal. In the 1890s, Dr. John Harvey Kellogg, along with his younger brother Will, invented corn flakes by accident while trying to create a healthy cracker to serve Kellogg's patients. While John Harvey resisted it, Will began coating corn flakes in sugar and pitched the processed food to the public as a healthy alternative to the typical American breakfast of eggs, bacon, and potatoes. Within a few years, Will K. Kellogg had purchased the rights to corn flakes from his older brother and formed the "Battle Creek Toasted Corn Flake Company" (known today as Kellogg's).[1] Eventually, Kellogg's was spurred by new competition to abandon their health angle, and instead created cereals that focused on taste and convenience. The end result was processed wheat, corn, and oat products laced with increasing amounts of sugar. (It was like a sweetener arms race.) Kellogg's Corn Flakes inspired Cheerios, which gave way to Honey Nut Cheerios. Froot Loops led to Lucky Charms, which led to Chocolate Lucky Charms and Lucky Charms Frosted Flakes. There are Cookie Crisp, Cinnamon Toast Crunch, Trix, and countless other cereals that feature cartoon characters, dessert ingredients, and spoonfuls of sugar.

And, I've got a confession: I've always loved cereal. As a child, I ate bowl after bowl of sugary cereals. When I grew up, I ate Fiber One on top of my yogurt while sitting in my cubicle at work. I thought it was very healthy for my body (because all that fiber would help me lose weight) and just didn't understand why I didn't look and feel my best after eating it.

Now I understand why a big bowl of cereal made me feel crummy. That's because most cereals are highly processed food products, chock full of questionable ingredients like BHT, artificial colors, cellulose, and GMO ingredients. In addition, they're almost always full of sugar—typically one of the first ingredients—which can lead to a massive spike in blood sugar, followed by a crash soon after. This is especially true of cereals aimed at children.

On the one hand, it's *crazy* that Big Food has convinced parents it's okay to feed their children processed foods like this for breakfast. You'd never give your child a bowl of marshmallows or cookies for breakfast, so why would you give them a bowl of Lucky Charms or Cookie Crisp? It makes no sense.

How did Big Food persuade parents that sugary cereals are a suitable breakfast? One of their key marketing tricks was to fortify breakfast cereal with vitamins. Lucky Charms might have lots of sugary marshmallows, but it also has a slew of vitamins and minerals that are added artificially and highlighted on the box. As a result, parents give in when their children ask for the "magically delicious" cereal. Anything with 25 percent of your recommended daily allowance for all those vitamins can't be *that* bad for you, can it?

This chapter is about how the fortification lie has been used to con us into thinking junk food is an acceptable meal. Because as you'll soon see, the problems with fortification go way beyond breakfast cereal.

Imagine the following scenario: You're on your weekly grocery shopping trip. You reach for an energy drink with a label that features, in a large font, "Now with ginkgo biloba." You're not sure exactly what gingko biloba is, but your best friend swears by its magical ability to improve memory. It's a little pricey at $2.99 for 12 ounces, but you decide that it's still a pretty cheap price to pay for brain health. You don't give the purchase a second thought.

The truth is, you should. That drink is an example of a fortified food product, and they crowd grocery store shelves and confuse consumers.

Food makers pack products with vitamins, minerals, herbs, and other nutrients to try to make them seem healthier than they really are. This is called food fortification. It is designed to trick us into thinking a food is good for us because it has been fortified—but the idea that fortified food is automatically healthy is a lie.

For one thing, most fortified foods are processed, so fortified junk food is still junk food. The addition of vitamins and minerals to the food product does nothing to absolve these foods of their sins of added sugars, excess sodium, artificial flavorings, dyes, inflammatory fats, processed starches, and preservatives.

WHY THE LIE?

For perspective, fortification wasn't always a food lie. The practice of fortifying foods started a long time ago—and with good and honorable intentions.

It was 1921. During an American Medical Association convention, two Akron, Ohio, doctors addressed a raging health problem in certain areas of the U.S., enlarged thyroid glands—a condition better known as goiter. In a clinical trial, the doctors discovered that iodine treatments prevented goiter in Akron schoolgirls.[2] When the body didn't have enough iodine, it was unable to properly synthesize thyroid hormones. This can cause unsightly neck goiters. Iodine deficiency is generally found in regions where the iodine in soil has dwindled because of floods or heavy rainfall, or if the area was once covered by glaciers.[3]

Prior to the Akron study, research from Europe had also found an association between iodine deficiency and goiter. Public health officials in the U.S. were galvanized and eager to act. By May 1, 1924 the Morton Salt Company was distributing the "goiter cure" to households nationwide: iodized salt. It was the first time a vitamin or mineral deficiency was corrected through people's food—a practice we now call food fortification.

Several major waves of food fortification followed: milk was fortified with vitamin D in the 1930s, wheat flour became enriched specific nutrients (niacin, iron, thiamin, and riboflavin) in the 1940s; calcium was added to a several food products beginning in the 1980s,[4] followed by the addition of folic acid in the 1990s to enriched grain products after several studies found that the nutrient could help reduce neural tube defects in newborns.[5] Now, you find calcium-fortified juice, omega-3 fortified bread, and many other fortified food products lining the aisles of every major grocery store.

The upshot of all this is that foods are increasingly turning into dietary supplements, drugs, or something in between. Once we had orange juice. Now we have orange juice with added calcium. Once we had pea soup. Then we had pea soup with added St. John's wort. Once we had bottled water. Then we had Vitaminwater. Now, we've even got bottled water with added protein. What's going on with our food supply?

Profits, that's what. Food manufacturers and marketers have identified herbs, minerals, vitamins, and other nutrients that come with potential benefits. And, for better or for worse, they are mining those ingredients to create and advertise more fortified foods and "functional foods."

Although fortification may have started out with good intentions, today manufacturers use it to push their products and drive sales, sometimes using excessive amounts that aren't particularly safe (especially for young children). Worst of all, fortification is often used to sell food that isn't good for us.

THE TRUTH ABOUT FOOD FORTIFICATION

In some cases, the benefits are welcome. If you don't drink milk or eat dairy foods, orange juice fortified with calcium sounds like it'd be beneficial. If you're ready to get pregnant, whole grains fortified with folic acid seem to make good sense.

But problems arise when the added substances haven't been adequately tested to make sure they're safe, or when the purported benefit is based on little or no evidence, or when only a trivial amount of a beneficial ingredient is added, or when you replace healthy foods like fruits and vegetables with fortified candy bars, chips, sodas, teas, and other junk foods. I maintain that this "value"-added grub, which is sometimes sold at a premium price, deceives and bilks you by dangling the promise of unproven health benefits made by companies interested in only boosting their profits at your expense.

And if you eat processed foods (especially bread, snack bars, cereals, wheat pasta, and nutritional shakes), it's nearly impossible to avoid synthetic vitamins. Synthetic vitamins are made in labs using raw materials such as coal tar, corn sugars, petroleum, or acetylene gas.[6] During the processing, these materials are exposed to other chemicals and extremely high temperatures.

Furthermore, there's suggestive evidence that the body absorbs these synthetic nutrients differently from natural nutrients. Studies have found, for instance, that naturally occurring vitamin E (such as is found in avocados, for instance) is absorbed by the body about twice as efficiently as synthetic vitamin E.[7] It's unclear why that might be, but one likely possibility is that whole foods also provide important enzymes, minerals, and cofactors that make it easier for us to metabolize vitamins.[8]

The science behind fortified and functional foods remains flimsy because it takes a lot of money and resources to prove that a nutrient or food ingredient really prevents or cures a disease.

Are Nutrition Facts Really "Facts"?

All food companies are required to have a Nutrition Facts label on their package—you know, the one that lists out how many calories, fat grams, and nutrients the product contains. The problem? These "facts" aren't always telling the truth.

You see, government regulations allow a margin of error of 20 percent.[9] So that product with 100 percent of the daily recommendation for vitamin A might really contain 120 percent. That 100-calorie pack of cookies could really be 120 calories. While this may seem minor, it could really add up for people who need to closely watch their consumption of certain nutrients, or sodium, for instance.

Conversely, some products may contain less of the nutrients than the Nutrition Facts label states. When the U.S. Government Accountability Office audited certain food products, they found that a third of them were inaccurate in regard to iron content and almost half of them had the wrong vitamin A content listed.[10] This leaves open the possibility that companies could label their products as containing 15 percent of recommended iron (or another nutrient) when it truly doesn't contain any, and still remain within the law.

The solution? Don't bother relying on the Nutrition Facts panel to ensure you're meeting nutrient needs. Instead, focus on eating whole, real food that doesn't need a label saying it's healthy.

ACTION STEPS: CHOOSE FORTIFIED FOODS WISELY

BE SURE YOU'RE NOT OD-ING ON VITAMINS AND MINERALS.

Fortified foods are cleverly marketed to moms and dads who want to make sure their children are getting enough vitamins and minerals. But there's a hitch. The Environmental Working Group, a nonprofit health research and advocacy group, analyzed the vitamin and mineral content of 1,550 brands of cereal. Out of those, they found that 114 of them were actually fortified with excessive amounts of vitamin A, zinc, or niacin. The guilty cereals include some that you may even have in your kitchen cabinets right now: Kellogg's Krave, Total Raisin Bran, Smart Start, and Cocoa Krispies. Likewise, they evaluated 1,000 different snack bars and found 27 of them that are over-fortified. Some of the worst offenders were Balance, KIND, and Marathon bars.[11]

This could easily become a problem if someone eats a few servings of fortified foods each day, as children often do in America. The EWG concluded that "up to half of young children get too much of vitamin A, zinc, and niacin" due to fortified foods. Overdosing on these nutrients over time can lead to some health issues, such as liver damage, skeletal abnormalities, osteoporosis, and impaired copper absorption. The EWG also advised that pregnant women especially monitor their intake of fortified foods, because they are commonly already taking prenatal vitamin supplements and too much vitamin A is associated with birth defects.

Along the same lines, calcium is being added to more and more foods; it's more than possible to inadvertently get far more than the recommended 1,000 to 1,200 milligrams a day—especially if you also take a mineral supplement. High doses of supplemental calcium may increase the risk of kidney stones. On the other hand, foods naturally rich in calcium seem to protect against kidney stones. Crazy, right?

The moral of the story: it's best to obtain your vitamins and minerals in a natural state—and that means from whole foods.

For This Nutrient:	Eat Naturally Occurring Sources:	Rather Than:
Thiamin (B$_1$)	Trout, lean pork, whole-grain bread, sunflower seeds, acorn squash, peas	White bread, processed cereals
Riboflavin (B$_2$)	Yogurt, mushrooms, spinach, almonds, lean meats	White bread, processed cereals
Niacin (B$_3$)	Yellowfin tuna, lean meats, peanuts, portobello mushrooms, sunflower seeds, peas, avocado	White bread, processed cereals
Folic Acid (B$_9$)	Black beans, lentils, spinach, asparagus, sunflower seeds, Romaine lettuce, broccoli, turnip greens, mango, peanuts, fresh squeezed orange juice, whole-grain bread	White bread, processed cereals
Vitamin C	Yellow bell peppers, guava, kale, kiwi, broccoli, citrus fruits, berries	Fortified orange juice
Vitamin D	Mushrooms, oily fish, tofu, eggs	Fortified cereals, milk, soy milk, orange juice, and cereals
Calcium	Dark leafy greens, mozzarella cheese, yogurt, bok choy, okra, broccoli, almonds	Fortified soy foods, tofu that is prepared with calcium sulfate, calcium-fortified orange juice, some bottled waters and energy bars
Iron	Squash, pumpkin seeds, shellfish, nuts, lean red meat, white beans, lentils, dark leafy greens	Fortified cereals

Don't go overboard with omega-3s.

Omega-3 fatty acids—those super-healthy fats we get naturally from fish and some vegetables—are popping up in food and beverages like crazy. They're being added to breads, spreads, cereals, baby formula, protein powers, frozen waffles, and even pasta and cheese.

We definitely need omega-3s in our diets. According to research, omega-3 fats can help numerous conditions: heart disease, high blood pressure, type 2 diabetes, obesity, inflammatory diseases, brain disorders, and vision problems.[12]

Fortifying foods with these fats may sound like a good idea, especially if you don't eat fish. But is fortifying food with omega-3s versus obtaining it from natural sources the healthiest way to go?

I contend that it's still best to get your omega-3s from whole foods, such as wild-caught fish. Let me tell you why:

Most fortified foods provide only a fraction of what's recommended for potential benefits. A cup of fortified orange juice, for example, may have 50 milligrams of the two main omega-3s (EPA and DHA), which is virtually nothing compared to salmon. Fortified products often cost more too. That fortified orange juice is not much more than a marketing ploy to get you to buy it.

Omega-3 fortified products are not necessarily healthy. A cup of Horizon Organic Lowfat Chocolate Milk with DHA omega-3, for example, has 27 grams of sugar. Fortified granola bars may contain a lot of sugar too. They're even adding omega-3s to sugary breakfast cereal, as if a smidgen of fortification can make up for the big dose of sugar and heavily processed ingredients.

That's why I believe it's always better to get your nutrients from whole food. As for omega-3s from natural sources, here are my top 10 picks:

1. Mackerel
2. Salmon (wild caught)
3. Walnuts
4. Chia seeds

5. Herring

6. Hemp seeds

7. Flaxseeds (ground) or flaxseed oil

8. Tuna

9. White fish

10. Spinach

BEWARE OF HERBAL FORTIFICATION.

Increasingly, food companies are fortifying their products with medicinal herbs. Is this bad? After all, herbs have been used by humans for thousands of years to maintain health and treat diseases—and in my experience, they offer a viable alternative to treatment with prescription drugs.

But it's important to be clear-eyed about these medicinal herbs that are being used and abused by Big Food. In general, I see the fortification of food and beverages with herbs largely as a lure to get health-conscious consumers to spend more money. In other words, it's yet another marketing ploy, meant to sway us into believing that processed food products are healthier than real foods, which they are not.

You find added herbs mostly in beverages. For instance, take PepsiCo's line of fruity herb-fortified drinks SoBe, which are infused with a blend of guarana, ginseng, yerba mate, hibiscus, chamomile, and rose hips. That sounds healthy, right? What's less obvious is that a 20-ounce bottle of SoBe also contains upward of 63 grams of sugar. In other words, the herbs provide a halo of health to an otherwise toxic product.

But even if you choose an herbal product that doesn't contain lots of sugar, there are still some safety concerns and you could put yourself at risk for potential herb-drug interactions. Some herbs can affect the metabolism of drugs, increasing their action too much, or otherwise interfere with them.

The chart below highlights some major herb-drug interactions.

Herb	Drugs	Interactions
Echinacea	Immunosuppressants and corticosteroids	The herb can stop these drugs from working properly because it stimulates the immune system.
Ephedra	MAO inhibitors (a class of antidepressants)	Increases the risk of high blood pressure, even coma.
Garlic	Blood thinners; diabetes medication	Garlic can increase abnormal bleeding and interfere with medication designed to lower blood sugar.
Gingko biloba	Blood-thinner agents; blood pressure medication	This combo may increase the risk of bleeding, and reduce the effectiveness of blood pressure drugs. (Gingko interacts with nearly 500 drugs.)
Ginseng	Diabetes medications; blood thinners	This combo may result in hypoglycemia (abnormally low blood sugar); may decrease the effectiveness of blood thinners, increasing the risk of clotting.
Kava kava	Anti-anxiety drugs	This can overly increase sedation.
Licorice	Prednisone	Increases the effects of steroid drugs.
St. John's wort	Antidepressants; sedatives	Increases the risk of "serotonin syndrome," a potentially fatal condition that occurs when drug or herb interactions cause the brain chemical serotonin to increase to dangerous levels.

Protect yourself from potential interactions if you take herbs, whether in food or beverages or as supplements. Always consult your pharmacist or physician before taking any herbs, especially if you are also on medications, if you are pregnant, or within two weeks of surgery.

MAKE HEALTHY PROBIOTIC CHOICES.

When I was younger, I was plagued with stomach problems. I suffered from painful tummy aches half an hour or so after eating, leaving me feeling uncomfortable, crampy, and bloated. On a bad night I'd be kept awake until the wee hours with a bubbling, churning sensation in my stomach. I sometimes missed school because of how awful I felt. As a kid, this seemed to me like the end of the world.

What I didn't know then was that my diet of Lunchables, microwaveable cheese sticks, fast food, and candy was destroying healthy bacteria in my gut. Those little bacterial warriors (probiotics) are super important to overall health. Among their long list of good deeds, beneficial bacteria in the gut help keep your immune and digestive systems strong. I was filling up on sugar, refined carbs, food additives, and junk foods—which were emptying my body of exactly what I needed to help with my digestive issues!

In order to foster healthy bacteria in the gut, you need to give them the perfect environment to thrive. And most of them don't care for processed foods and junk foods; they prefer "prebiotics," which are basically soluble fibers found in many natural foods such as the Jerusalem artichoke, garlic, rye, banana, and onion.

Without the right nutrition, the gut is damaged. There's evidence that fats, salt, and refined sugar, consumed in excess, along with additives and toxins in processed foods, may lead to leaky gut syndrome—which creates tiny little holes in our digestive system organs that leak out the good bacteria we need to stay healthy and keep our immune system strong.[13] A leaky gut puts you at risk[14] for inflammatory bowel disease, asthma, food allergies, arthritis, celiac disease, and even cancer. An animal study conducted at Thomas Jefferson University identified a substance in the intestines that prevents cancer by acting as a tumor suppressor.[15] Without it, the intestinal barrier weakens, allowing cancerous agents to "leak" into other parts of the body, which can lead to occurrences of cancer beyond the intestine (in the liver, lung, and lymph nodes).

All along, my childhood diet—high in sugar and fat and low in fiber—was making my intestines porous with a leaky lining. It wasn't until I learned about the processed food industry and began eating real, nutritious food that these problems disappeared. I had no idea at the time—nobody did—but my processed food diet was causing inflammation and harming healthy gut bacteria. If only I knew then what I know now!

I bring this up because these days food companies are fortifying processed foods with probiotics. Yep, food products with these healthy bugs: non-fermented, probiotic-fortified tortilla chips, bread, and juice. It's a huge trend: tons of new packaged foods are being marketed as probiotic powerhouses, with the ability to colonize your gut with the healthy bacteria shown in research studies to help you lose weight, fight infection, and prevent disease.

I realize this sounds good, but here's the problem: When you scarf down a bowl of probiotic-fortified cereal that's full of sugar, you are still eating a ton of sugar. That sugar is not good for your gut flora, and could very well be cancelling out any benefits you might glean from the small amount of probiotics in the cereal. To date, there are no properly controlled studies about whether these processed foods with added probiotics can do anything for you. White bread with a probiotic is still white bread. So why spend your money?

If you want to improve your gut health, do it naturally. Limit sugar, refined grains, and refined oils, and eat fermented foods that naturally contain probiotics (such as plain organic yogurt, miso paste, tempeh, kimchi, kefir, and kombucha), and possibly take a high-quality probiotic supplement. Ever since I started adding fermented foods to my diet, I've gotten sick much less often. My stomach problems are in the past.

Also important: If you heat probiotic food, it kills the active cultures, rendering them useless. So keep this in mind when you're cooking with a probiotic-fortified food.

BE CHOOSY ABOUT CEREAL.

I know that, one day soon, my young daughter is going to ask me to buy one of those sugary cereals that line the cereal aisle. And I understand the temptation, both for children and parents. Healthy whole foods, after all, don't get cartoon characters, brightly colored bites, and big advertising budgets. And when parents are rushing in the morning, trying to get everyone off to school and work, it can be tempting to just pour some Lucky Charms in a bowl and call it a meal.

But I want my daughter to understand why these Big Food products aren't good for her, even if they're fortified with vitamins. I want to show her that it's possible to eat a healthy breakfast that's also delicious and easy to prepare, whether it's eggs and whole-grain toast; or oatmeal with fruit, nuts and a little maple syrup; or a yogurt parfait. These foods only take a few minutes to prepare and can often be prepped in advance, but I promise they'll make you and your family feel far better during the day.

And if she really wants cereal, or if we just don't have time for anything else in the morning, it's good to know there are some healthy cereals. The key is to look for cereals that contain nutritious ingredients, such as seeds, nuts, and dried fruit, and that are minimally processed. A few of my favorite cereals are:

> **Two Moms in the Raw Cereal:** This grain-free cereal is full of healthy fruit and nuts like almonds, walnuts, bananas, coconut, and dates.

> **Food for Life Ezekiel 4:9 Sprouted Grain Cereal:** The grains in this cereal are whole and sprouted, so they are easier for your body to digest and won't spike your blood sugar like flour-based cereal grains do. My favorite is their cinnamon raisin flavor.

One Degree Sprouted Brown Rice Crisps or Erewhon Crispy Brown Rice Cereal: Either of these makes an excellent replacement for Kellogg's Rice Krispies.

Qi'a Superfood Cereals: I love these blends of whole ingredients like buckwheat groats, chia seeds, hemp seeds, dried cranberries, and almonds. This cereal is delicious mixed with organic yogurt and fruit.

Purely Elizabeth Ancient Grain Granola: Comes in four different flavors: original, cranberry pecan, pumpkin fig, and blueberry hemp, made with healthy ingredients like quinoa, amaranth, chia seeds, and raw virgin coconut oil.

Chiarezza Almighty Mango Goji Cereal: Made from organic chia, hemp seeds, mango, buckwheat, banana flakes, and goji berries. As there are chia seeds in this one, you can also make a yummy pudding by pouring nut milk over it and letting it sit in the fridge for about 25 minutes.

Given a choice, I will always choose real food that is endowed by nature with vitamins and minerals rather than nutrient-fortified junk food. While it is important in some cases to rely on fortified food, in other cases, it's just another deceptive marketing tactic—or what Dr. David Katz calls "the nutritional equivalent of lipstick on a pig."[16]

CHAPTER 10

Weed Killer for Dinner

I want to be as clear as possible at the start of this chapter, because my words on genetically modified (GMO) foods have been twisted for years.

I am not fundamentally against biotechnology. I'm not even necessarily against all GMO food, although I acknowledge that certain experts stress how much uncertainty remains about their safety. As was noted by researchers at New York University, genetically modified foods (also known as GMOs, or genetically modified organisms) represent a massive experiment conducted on nature.[1] I believe companies pushing such products should present clear evidence that they are not causing harm, either to people or to the ecosystems we depend upon. Companies should also clearly label their food products so consumers are informed that they contain GMOs. If that position makes me a radical, then so be it. To me, it feels like common sense.

However, what I am strongly against are the chemicals that almost always go hand in hand with genetically modified crops. This chapter will focus on one of the main chemicals used during the farming of GMOs: Roundup weed killer, a mixture of glyphosate and surfactants. (You likely even have a bottle of this in your garage, as it's the world's most popular weed killer.) For years, Monsanto—the giant industrial agriculture company—has sold Roundup to farmers and consumers around the world. Genetically modified (GMO) versions of certain crops (corn, soy, sugar beets, canola, and more) have been developed to withstand being sprayed directly with Roundup weed killer. These GMO crops are called "Roundup-Ready."

What many people don't know, however, is that Roundup is also used on non-GMO crops such as wheat, where it is used to dry the crop 7 to 10 days before harvest. This is a problematic practice because spraying crops so close to harvest increases the amount of glyphosate incorporated into the food supply. It's not just the wheat. Roundup is used on major conventional non-GMO food crops such as tomatoes, nuts, oranges, and beans (upwards of 70 different food crops in the U.S.).[2] While most food products have never been tested for this weed killer's residue, as we'll learn later in this chapter, the tests that have been performed suggest that the majority of processed food sold in this country is contaminated with some level of glyphosate.

In recent decades, the use of Roundup has gone up exponentially, increasing 15-fold since Roundup-Ready GMO crops were introduced.[3] In fact, Roundup has become so popular that economists have started referring to it as "agricultural heroin" because many farmers are so addicted to it.

One of the problems with addictions is that, over time, you need to take higher doses to get the same effect. One drink becomes three, which becomes five. The same thing is happening with Roundup. As weeds develop resistance to the herbicide, farmers need to increase the amount of Roundup they spray on their fields.[4] That's great for Monsanto—they sell more weed killer—but, as you'll soon learn, really bad for us.

Roundup works because it contains glyphosate, a chemical first patented to remove mineral deposits from metal pipes. As you can probably guess, glyphosate is not a chemical you want in your body. That's because it works by disrupting a class of enzymes that are in virtually every living thing, from common weeds to human beings. These enzymes perform a wide variety of basic biological functions, one of which is removing toxins from your body. (This means that glyphosate can make us more vulnerable to other chemicals as well.)

But wait: it gets worse. Much worse. Glyphosate is also considered an "endocrine disruptor." Endocrine disruptors mimic or block the action of natural hormones and wreak havoc with your endocrine system (having a profoundly negative effect on the body). When you ingest endocrine disruptors, you are in essence altering your body's basic chemistry.[5]

One of the most damaging effects of glyphosate is that it stimulates overproduction of estrogen. This in turn can fuel the growth of estrogen-dependent breast cancer—a fact uncovered when researchers found the risk of breast cancer was even greater in those exposed to glyphosate who supplemented their diet with soybeans (also known to stimulate estrogen).[6]

Last but not least, there is increasing evidence that glyphosate can screw up the health of your gut microbiome, the community of bacteria and microorganisms that are key to a healthy digestive system.[7] This has led some scientists to speculate that the rise of weed killer is partially responsible for the growing incidence of a wide variety of gastrointestinal disorders, including celiac disease, gluten intolerance, and irritable bowel syndrome.

But don't take my word for it. Dave Schubert, Ph.D., head of the Salk Institute's Cellular Neurobiology Laboratory, puts it this way: "There is indeed an enormous amount of published data showing that Roundup is very nasty stuff, particularly at the levels currently being used (ten times more than before genetically modified, herbicide-resistant crops) and the extent of human exposure in food—a greatly allowed increase by the EPA to reflect increased use."[8]

To prove his point, Schubert cites studies documenting increases in cancer in farming areas of Argentina since the introduction of GMO crops and spikes in cancer in lab animals after exposure to GMO corn sprayed with the weed killer.

MONSANTO'S GUILT BEHIND CLOSED DOORS

Even Monsanto's own scientists and consultants have questioned the safety of glyphosate, but you won't find that in a company press release. In the late 1990s, Dr. James Parry, a Monsanto consultant, concluded that glyphosate is capable of producing genotoxicity (which is an adverse effect on cells that may lead to cancer).[9] But instead of listening to his concerns, Monsanto executives suppressed his findings and decided to seek out other consultants who were better at working with industry and helping them influence regulators. In one e-mail, a Monsanto executive admits that "we simply aren't going to do the studies Parry suggests" that would further examine the hazards of glyphosate.[10] (Sure seems to me they were scared of learning the truth.) In 2003, Monsanto toxicologist Donna Farmer warned company executives that they "cannot say that Roundup is not a carcinogen... we have not done the necessary testing on the formulation to make that statement."[11] Fifteen years later, they still haven't. And, neither has the EPA.[12]

WORLD HEALTH ORGANIZATION VERSUS MONSANTO

Meanwhile, the independent evidence linking Roundup's active ingredient, glyphosate, to serious health problems has only grown. In fact, the evidence is so persuasive that in March 2015 the World Health Organization's team of international cancer experts deemed glyphosate a "probable human carcinogen."[13] As could be expected, this expert panel, known as the International Agency for Research on Cancer (IARC), has been forced to defend ruthless attacks from the agrochemical industry since this finding. The industry has discredited their credibility in the media and even lobbied our government to take away their funding.[14] As we have seen throughout this book, the industry plays dirty when the truth comes out.

In January of 2018, IARC responded to this affront to their work: "Since the evaluation of glyphosate by the IARC Monographs Program in March 2015, the Agency has been subject to unprecedented, coordinated efforts to undermine the evaluation, the program and the organization. These efforts have deliberately and repeatedly misrepresented the Agency's work. The attacks have largely originated from the agro-chemical industry and associated media outlets."[15]

IARC went on to defend their position with respect to how they came to their conclusions on glyphosate and properly handled the data. They also provided substantial reasoning for why they only used publicly available research in their evaluation and confirmed that their members are free from conflict of interest.

This group of elite independent experts is standing firm in their convictions, yet many IARC members have felt stunned and intimidated by the industry's disruptive actions toward them. As one member of the panel, Francesco Forastiere, an Italian researcher specializing in epidemiology, put it, "We were not expecting this strong reaction and what happened. We were doing our job. We understood there were other issues . . . economic consequences. But none of us had a political agenda. We simply acted as scientists, evaluating the body of evidence, according to the IARC criteria."[16]

Yes, Dr. Forastiere hit the nail on the head. Those "economic consequences" mean a possible end to the industry's top billion-dollar weed killer. The stakes are high.

CORRUPTION AT ITS FINEST

Monsanto (and the agrochemical industry in general) responds to troubling evidence about Roundup in various ways. By shutting down additional research. By attacking those (like me) who dare to write about the evidence against Roundup. By funding front groups and paying for online trolls. By spending millions of dollars lobbying the government.

And, unfortunately, to some extent it's working.

In 2013, the EPA increased the industry standard of what is considered a "safe" level of glyphosate on our food[17] in order to make ever-growing amounts seem acceptable. Instead of properly regulating this probable carcinogen, they effectively raised the "safe" level in our food so that no one can blame the industry for poisoning us with unlawful amounts of chemicals. This is corruption at its finest.

Why did the EPA act this way? Some recently released internal e-mails between the EPA and Monsanto offer some tantalizing clues. (The e-mails were released as part of an ongoing class-action lawsuit alleging that exposure to Roundup can cause non-Hodgkin's lymphoma, which found that Monsanto was liable for $298 million because they knowingly concealed the risks.[18]) What the e-mails reveal is a close working relationship between high-level EPA officials and Monsanto. Jess Rowland, the official who was in charge of evaluating the cancer risk of glyphosate for the EPA, was allegedly helping Monsanto prevent another federal agency from investigating whether glyphosate causes cancer. Rowland even told a Monsanto employee, "If I can kill this I should get a medal."[19] Monsanto apparently agreed, as the company employees proposed hiring Rowland after he retired from the EPA.

Other e-mails show that Monsanto proposed ghostwriting a key report used by the EPA to evaluate glyphosate and just having the scientists sign their names to it. The crooked relationship between the EPA and Monsanto led some EPA officials to speak up. EPA toxicologist Marion, for instance, concluded, "It is essentially certain that glyphosate causes cancer," while criticizing Rowland for playing "political conniving games with the science." She pleaded with him, "For once do the right thing and don't make decisions based on how it affects your bonus."[20]

The EPA continues to pander to Monsanto. In late 2017 they declared their position that glyphosate is "not likely to be carcinogenic to humans," contradicting the World Health Organization IARC's findings.[21]

It's time for the EPA to put the public health above the corrupt desires of corporations.

WHY THE LIE?

Why does Big Food insist on suppressing the truth about its weed killer?

The obvious answer is money: Monsanto makes billions of dollars every year selling its herbicides to farmers, along with GMO seeds that are used in conjunction with these chemicals. They're terrified that if people learned the truth about glyphosate, we'd insist on foods grown without it.

But there's another reason: glyphosate has already contaminated our food supply. It's in countless food products. Big Food is worried that if we realized we were ingesting weed killer with our breakfast cereal, crackers, cookies, and chips, we'd be justifiably upset. It's much easier to not test for these toxins. Ignorance is bliss, at least when it comes to processed food.

Fortunately, we can take matters into our own hands. Not long ago, the grassroots advocacy group Food Democracy Now! issued a shocking report that showed just how prevalent Roundup is in our food.[22] They commissioned Anresco Laboratories, an FDA-registered food safety laboratory that's been around since 1943, to test popular U.S. food products for glyphosate residues. It was the first-ever independent analysis of glyphosate contamination in major American food brands. The results clearly showed that millions of people are being exposed to glyphosate on a daily basis. That's because the weed killer was found in iconic processed foods like Cheerios, Ritz Crackers, and Oreos.

Even if you don't personally eat the specific brands that were tested (and I don't), how many Americans are consuming these foods every day? How many of your friends and family have their cabinets filled with these famous brands? Would they still buy these foods if they knew tests found weed killer in them?

In case you're skeptical of relying on this one report, the Canadian government recently tested 3,188 food products. They found glyphosate residues in nearly 30 percent of them, including 36.6 percent of grain products and 31 percent of baby foods.[23] And the one time the United States government tested soybean samples, they found that 271 out of 300 had measurable levels of glyphosate residue.[24] Likewise, Carey Gillam, research director for U.S. Right to Know (a nonprofit consumer education group), reported that internal documents show the FDA has found glyphosate residues in infant oat cereal and honey samples—two foods that seem so innocuous.[25] The levels found in the honey exceeded regulatory limits in the European Union.

And this is just the start: There are still thousands of other brands and foods that have not been tested for glyphosate residues. The tragic truth is that glyphosate is so rampant in our food supply that Americans are effectively being forced to eat this poison. And yes, I said *poison*.

Glyphosate is really good at killing weeds.

It might also be killing us.

ACTION STEPS: GO ORGANIC ABOVE ALL

The best way to avoid glyphosate is by choosing Certified Organic foods because it is prohibited on organic crops. Although contamination is a real threat, from what we've seen in testing so far, the levels on organic foods are generally minimal compared to what's been found on conventional (nonorganic) foods. It's been shown that people who eat organic foods have less glyphosate and other synthetic pesticides in their systems.

STAY AWARE AND INFORMED!

This chapter is my perspective on GMOs and the chemicals that are used along with them, based on my years of research and investigation. I don't want to tell you how to think; I just want you to be aware of the lies and misinformation that exist on this subject. Ultimately, it's up to you to make your own food decisions. While more independent research is certainly needed, I've decided that when it comes to the health of my family and me, the risk of GMOs and glyphosate just isn't worth it.

CHAPTER 11

Organic
Deception

In the late 1940s, publisher J. I. Rodale decided to become a farmer. He'd spent most of his life in New York City, but he'd become increasingly interested in farming methods that didn't rely on toxic pesticides or big doses of nitrogen fertilizer. Although this "old-fashioned" style of farming had been the norm a few generations before, it had been largely replaced by industrial techniques that promised farmers higher yields and less labor.[1]

Unfortunately, these new agricultural techniques soon created some major problems. During the Second World War, for instance, farmers were no longer able to buy their chemical fertilizers, since those same chemicals were needed to make munitions for the army. (They also required vast amounts of energy to produce, but that's another story.) The shortfall of chemicals revealed the destructive impact of even a few decades of industrial agriculture, as farmers were forced to deal with the sudden "nutrient poverty" of their soil. While old-fashioned farming techniques helped maintain a healthy topsoil, industrial methods depended on a steady influx of chemicals. Take away those chemicals and harvests plummet.

Rodale wanted to start a farm that could preserve "old school" chemical-free farming techniques. (He'd been influenced by British pioneers like Albert Howard and Lady Eve Balfour.)

"Organics is not a fad," Rodale wrote in 1954. "It has been a long-established practice—much more firmly grounded than the current chemical flair. Present agricultural practices are leading us downhill."[2] And so Rodale founded a 333-acre farm in rural Pennsylvania that featured livestock (for manure), composting, multiple crops with crop rotations, and various chemical-free techniques that kept the soil healthy and reduced the chemical load. One of Rodale's fundamental insights was that healthy living required a healthy agricultural system. If the dirt was full of poisons, our food would be full of poisons too.

Since Rodale helped start organic farming in America, his small experiment has become a major growth industry, with organic food accounting for roughly 5 percent of the total American food market. A few years ago, we could buy organic apples and broccoli. Now most grocery stores stock a full array of organic items, from pasta to yogurt, coffee to cookies, grapes to kale.

With these new alternatives come hard choices. Each week, you stand in a supermarket aisle looking at the bins of lemons. To your right, there is a small selection of organic lemons; to your left, conventional mass-produced lemons. The first is significantly more expensive than the latter. And so you ask yourself: Is organic worth it? Should I be willing to pay significantly more money for food that's grown without pesticides and chemicals?

For me, the answer is a definite yes. I believe that buying quality organic food ultimately saves you money down the road in medical costs, prescription drugs, and doctor visits. After I switched to eating primarily organic foods, everything changed in my life. I went from being overweight and sick to feeling vibrant and healthy. My skin issues vanished. I was able to stop taking my prescription medications.

My own experience with organic food is why I feel so strongly that organic food is an essential feature of a healthy diet. I'm aware of the chemicals that are used in conventional farming, and I know how bad they are for our health and the environment. I also know how bad they make things taste.

I like the purity of strawberries that have not been sprayed with dozens of pesticides. I prefer meat that has not been laced with growth hormones and antibiotics or raised in cruel feedlots. Organic fruit may not always look as pretty, but it tastes better. (So do organic meat and chicken.) This is what food should be.

And it's also better for your health. Many of these chemicals can make you tired, destroy your gut, wreak havoc on your complexion, and cause mood issues. Even worse, they may put you at risk for terrifying, life-shortening diseases like cancer.

So when I eat organic food, I know I'm making the right choice for my health and my body. When I buy organic food, I know I'm doing something positive for the environment and for the farmers who grow food in a sustainable manner. When I serve organic food, I know I'm not feeding synthetic pesticides, GMOs, growth hormones, or antibiotics to my friends and family. When I go organic, I have peace of mind. For people like me, organic food is more than just a label: it's a lifestyle.

But not everyone agrees with me. Regardless of the truth, the conventional food and chemical industries have gone to great lengths to spread a dangerous lie. In short, they want us to believe that organic food is neither better nor healthier than conventional food, and that it's definitely not worth the extra expense. And they've gotten a lot of help from the media in broadly disseminating this lie:

> Buying organic veggies at the supermarket is a waste of money—Quartz[3]

> The USDA "Organic" Label Misleads and Rips Off Consumers—*Forbes*[4]

> . . . Organic Foods Are Just a "Marketing Label"—*Business Insider*[5]

> Don't Believe the (Organic) Hype—NPR[6]

> Is Organic Food Worth the Higher Price? Experts say "no"—*Portland Tribune*[7]

Who is really telling the story here? Remember that Big Food and Big Ag rely heavily on front groups to promote these types of messages in the media, and they even go as far as to train seemingly independent farmers, bloggers, and scientists to act as expert sources for journalists. It's an elaborate con that the media keeps falling for.

Because here's the truth: Big Food is waging a war against organic food, with the good guys being battered by industry front groups armed with millions of dollars from food and chemical companies. In 2015, the advocacy group Friends of the Earth produced a report called *Spinning Food: How Food Industry Front Groups and Covert Communications Are Shaping the Story of Food.*[8] Their report exposed the dirty tactics that Big Food and agrochemical companies have implemented to combat the organic food movement. It reveals how they are using their deep pockets to launch stealth public relations campaigns and push coordinated messages that attack organic food and activists like me. At the same time, these groups defend the continued use of synthetic pesticides, antibiotics, GMOs, and chemical food additives.

As was documented in this report, four of the largest food and chemical trade associations have spent insane amounts of money—over half a billion dollars from 2009 to 2013 (which includes, but isn't limited to, public relations activities). This just goes to show, they've got deep pockets! They also uncovered that 14 of the largest front groups working for the industry spent about $126 million during that same time period, often without fully disclosing where their funding comes from.

One of these industry groups, the Alliance for Food and Farming, is funded by conventional produce farmers. They continually attack EWG's Dirty Dozen Guide on pesticides in conventional produce. Other industry groups such as the Council for Biotechnology Information and the Coalition for Safe and Affordable Food advocate for GMOs (GMOs are banned in organic farming), while Keep Food Affordable advocates for conventional meat and egg producers.[9]

The Pork Network warned farmers about "Crunchy Mamas"—demonizing moms who prefer organic food and are concerned about the conditions on factory farms.[10] The BlogHer Publishing Network conferences (the largest women's blogging network in the country) have been sponsored by several Big Food companies and the front group CommonGround[11] in an apparent attempt to influence the content on their network of blogs. In 2014, Monsanto paid bloggers $150 to attend a brunch following the BlogHer conference to learn "how farmers are using fewer resources to feed a growing population."[12] When I spoke at BlogHer Food in May 2016, Monsanto and its PR firm were in the audience taking notes feverishly. As a female activist, I'm particularly disgusted with these attempts to try to undermine and discredit me and other female bloggers, especially mothers who are trying to change our unhealthy food system.

What should we do with this information?

If you believe in organic foods and farming, as I do, I recommend you familiarize yourself with the key PR players and front groups—and most importantly, share that information far and wide. All of us who are advocating for a safer food system are up against huge corporations (and shady front groups) capable of spending tens of millions of dollars to preserve the status quo, which is leading to skyrocketing rates of obesity, diabetes, and allergies. If we are going to get the truth out there, we all have to work together.

Organic Pop Quiz

How well versed are you in organic foods? Take this quick quiz to find out.

1. How can you tell the difference between organic and nonorganic foods?
    a. If one food smells fresher than another, it's organic.
    b. It bears an organic label.
    c. The organic variety will always cost more.
    d. There's no difference.

2. What portion of food must be organic to permit a food manufacturer to use the USDA Certified Organic seal?

    a. 10 percent or less

    b. 25 percent

    c. 25 to 75 percent

    d. 95 to 100 percent

3. To bear the organic label, a food cannot be produced with:

    a. Roundup weed killer

    b. GMOs

    c. Irradiation

    d. All of the above

4. Organic foods often cost more than conventional foods because of:

    a. Higher taxes to organic farmers

    b. Production costs

    c. Greed

5. Besides buying organic foods, you can avoid toxins and other harmful ingredients by:

    a. Eating a variety of fresh, nonpackaged foods, such as fresh fruit, vegetables, nuts, and seeds.

    b. Eating food that is labeled "natural" or "all natural."

    c. Eating food that is labeled "free of artificial ingredients."

6. Organic fish can be found in the supermarket.

    ❑ True

    ❑ False

7. For organic meat, the USDA standards require that animals are:

    a. Raised in conditions that accommodate their natural behaviors.

b. Given organic feed.

c. Not administered antibiotics or hormones.

d. All of the above.

Answers:

1. The correct answer is: *It bears an organic label.* The label will state "USDA Organic."

2. The correct answer is: *95 to 100 percent.* Foods with 95 percent or more organic ingredients can use the USDA Certified Organic label or label their product as organic.

3. The correct answer is: *All of the above.* This is the beauty of organic food; it is grown and manufactured without toxins and processes that are harmful to health.

4. The correct answer is: *Production costs.* Not as many organic ingredients are available. So companies that buy them may have to pay more for them. Organic farming also is more labor intensive, which often leads to smaller yields.

5. The correct answer is: *Eating a variety of fresh, non-packaged foods.* Labels on packaged foods like "natural," "all natural," and "free of artificial ingredients" can be misleading to consumers, as they may be made with conventionally grown crops sprayed with Roundup, and may still contain GMOs and controversial additives.

6. The correct answer is: *False.* The USDA has not yet determined standards for what would make fish organic. The best option for fish is "wild" versus "farmed" varieties.

7. The correct answer is: *All of the above.* This standard applies to organic eggs and milk as well.

WHY THE LIE?

The biggest perpetrators of lies about organic food are Monsanto and other big agrochemical companies, like Dow and Bayer. Think about it: Their best-selling products—Roundup, pesticides, and GMO seeds—are banned on organic farms. If all farms went organic, their most profitable products would disappear. Any messaging that organic food is better than conventionally grown food is thus harmful to their business, so they dig into their deep wallets to push back against the evidence and sow mistrust of organic farming. They don't want Americans to question where their food comes from, because that would threaten their fat profit margins.

In this chapter, I'm going to present the case for organic food, as well as address some of the longstanding lies about organic farming, so you can decide what is best for yourself and your family.

Understand What Non-GMO Means —It's Not the Same as Organic!

There's a lot of muddled information and debate about what non-GMO and organic labels really mean. The labels are very different! It's crucial to understand the difference if you want to pick out the healthiest and safest food for you and your family. Every time we decide to buy a product, we are supporting so much more than our bodies. We are helping shape the policies and priorities of the entire food system. And this is why I want you to understand what the "non-GMO" label means.

The Non-GMO Project offers a third-party verification service for food companies who want to label their products as non-GMO. If you're in the U.S. or Canada, I'm sure you've seen their "butterfly" non-GMO label on products at the store. This verification label indicates that the product undergoes ongoing testing of all at-risk ingredients and the manufacturer complies with rigorous traceability and segregation practices.

The Non-GMO Project verification is audited every year to ensure compliance.

That said, this is not the primary label that I look for on the food I buy. When I have a choice, I always choose Certified Organic foods instead. That's because organic beats non-GMO every time. Here's why:

- **Certified organic foods are also non-GMO.** USDA organic regulations prohibit any genetically modified (GMO) ingredients in a Certified Organic product.

- **Organic crops cannot be grown with synthetic pesticides, and contain much lower pesticide residues than conventional crops overall.** Organic regulations prohibit certain toxic pesticides from being used on crops, but there are no special restrictions for non-GMO crops. As a result, non-GMO crops can be grown the same way as other conventional crops and can still be laden with toxic pesticide residues, including organophosphates that are linked to lymphoma and leukemia.

- **The most widely used herbicide on the planet—Roundup—is prohibited on organic crops.** Non-GMO crops such as wheat can be treated pre-harvest with glyphosate.

- **Organic ingredients aren't processed with toxic hexane.** Most vegetable oils (canola, soybean, corn, sunflower) are extracted using the neurotoxin hexane (distilled from crude oil), and some residue may remain in these oils. Hexane is also used in the processing of many soy ingredients like soy protein and textured vegetable protein. There's nothing prohibiting hexane-processed ingredients in non-GMO products, but hexane is banned from production of USDA organic products.

- **Organic crops are prohibited from being fertilized with sewage sludge.** Conventional non-GMO crops can be treated with "biosolids," a polite term for the treated waste that's flushed down the toilet, along with waste from hospitals and industry. This waste can be contaminated with such things as heavy metals, endocrine disruptors, pathogens, pharmaceuticals, pesticides, and dioxins—it's basically a toxic chemical soup!

- **Organic meat isn't produced with risky growth-promoting drugs, such as ractopamine.** Packaged non-GMO foods may contain meat that has been raised on ractopamine.

- **Organic animals aren't fattened up with growth-promoting antibiotics.** Antibiotics aren't just used to fight infection in farm animals; they're also used to fatten them up. The overuse of growth-promoting antibiotics is creating superbugs that could threaten the entire human population. There is nothing prohibiting the use of antibiotics in non-GMO products containing meat.

THE TRUTH ABOUT ORGANIC FOOD

GREATER NUTRITION

Eating organic certainly does you no harm, but does it truly enhance your health? While the scientific data is a bit limited, several studies point to organic foods being significantly more nutritious. For example, researchers at the University of California, Davis analyzed organic tomatoes and found that they had higher levels of flavonoids than nonorganic tomatoes.[13] Another study published in *PLOS ONE* found organic tomatoes had more vitamin C and lycopene (an antioxidant).[14] And a 2014 statistical analysis published in the *British Journal of Nutrition* found up to 69 percent more antioxidants in organic foods versus their nonorganic counterparts.[15] These researchers also found that organic foods contain lower levels of the toxic heavy metal cadmium and pesticides. Another large 2016 analysis published in the same journal found greater amounts of beneficial omega-3 fatty acids (about 50 percent more!) in organic meat and dairy.[16] This is because organic animals typically dine on more grass than conventional factory-farm livestock, producing a healthier fatty-acid profile.

Yes, I'd like to see more studies like these. But limited scientific evidence doesn't mean we should deny the data that does exist. Furthermore, it's important to understand why there aren't more studies about the benefits of organic food. One main reason is that a lot of nutritional research is funded by those with anti-organic interests, especially the biotech, Big Ag, and food companies that don't produce organic food. Needless to say, these companies have no interest in paying for science that documents the inferiority of their products.

BETTER FOR THE WAISTLINE

Of course, the benefits of organic food aren't limited to additional nutrients: eating organically may also help you stay thin. Antibiotics, growth hormones, pesticides, and synthetic preservatives are just a few of the chemicals that researchers have defined as obesogens.[17] The theory that obesogens in our food and environment could be making us fat has been gathering steam ever since researcher Paula Baillie-Hamilton published an article in the *Journal of Alternative and Complementary Medicine* in 2002, presenting strong evidence that chemical exposure caused weight gain in experimental animals.[18] As was reported in a *New York Times* piece "Warnings from a Flabby Mouse," exposure to endocrine-disrupting chemicals can promote weight gain.[19] This is important because many of the synthetic pesticides found on conventional crops are endocrine disruptors. Minimizing your exposure to obesogens by choosing an organic diet may be the boost you need to lose weight and keep it off.

CLEANER INGREDIENTS LISTS

In my own experience, eating organic also makes it much easier to avoid those highly toxic processed foods that are so unhealthy for us. By choosing Certified Organic food, you'll automatically avoid many potentially dangerous food additives—like TBHQ, BHT, artificial sweeteners (aspartame, sucralose), and artificial food dyes (Yellow #5, etc.), which are all banned from Certified Organic products. Although you always need to read the ingredients list, even on organic products, with organics it's easier to find products without a crazy long list of additives and that actually contain real food.

PROTECT YOUR FAMILY FROM HARMFUL PESTICIDES

Eating organic foods helps you avoid a cocktail of synthetic chemical pesticides, including the herbicide Roundup (which we discussed in the last chapter). One of the most fascinating reports on the problem of pesticides comes from a large project commissioned by the European Parliament. Experts from around the world were asked to study whether organic food and farming are healthier for us—and their findings run counter to everything you may have heard about organic food in the media. Quoting the coauthor of the report, Philippe Grandjean, adjunct professor of environmental health at Harvard T. H. Chan School of Public Health, here are some of his conclusions:

- "In conventional food, there are pesticide residues that remain in the food even after it's washed. Organic foods are produced virtually without pesticides."

- "Three long-term birth cohort studies in the U.S. suggest that pesticides are harming children's brains. In these studies, researchers found that women's exposure to pesticides during pregnancy, measured through urine samples, was associated with negative impacts on their children's IQ and neurobehavioral development, as well as with ADHD diagnoses."

- "Although the scientific evidence on pesticides' impact on the developing brain is incomplete, pregnant and breastfeeding women, and women planning to become pregnant, may wish to eat organic foods as a precautionary measure because of the significant and possibly irreversible consequences for children's health."[20]

The fundamental goal of organic farming is to produce food without using toxic pesticides. Crops are managed in a way that prevents the need to use chemicals. When produce from farms has been tested, organic typically has far less pesticide residue than conventional (nonorganic). A 2014 review published in the *British Journal of Nutrition* found pesticide residues four times more frequently on conventional crops.[21] By eating organic, you can significantly decrease your exposure to these chemicals that were designed to destroy other living things.

Also, pesticide consumption can have a cumulative effect, both in the immediate and long term, says the Pesticide Action Network.[22] Over time, this can damage your kidneys and liver, both of which have to work extra hard to remove these poisons from your body. And it's not just your major organs: pesticides wreak havoc everywhere. In general, the consumption and overload of pesticides may contribute to a slew of health issues, including:

- Cancer
- Alzheimer's
- Parkinson's
- Type 2 diabetes
- Obesity
- Food allergies
- Infertility

Pesticides are even more damaging to children than adults. The damage starts in the womb—something corroborated by the American Academy of Pediatrics in the following statement:

> Epidemiologic evidence demonstrates associations between early life exposure to pesticides and pediatric cancers, decreased cognitive function, and behavioral problems. . . . Recognizing and reducing problematic exposures will require attention to current inadequacies in medical training, public health tracking, and regulatory action on pesticides. . . . For many children, diet

may be the most influential source, as illustrated by an intervention study that placed children on an organic diet (produced without most conventional pesticides) and observed drastic and immediate decrease in urinary excretion of organophosphate pesticide metabolites.[23]

SAFER FOR FARMERS

Let's not forget about the impact that conventional agriculture has on farmers. Tens of thousands of farmworkers are poisoned by pesticides each year in the U.S., according to EPA reports[24]—and there are likely many incidents that go unreported. The effects on farmers and nearby communities are devastating.

In 2010, the Department of Health and Human Services President's Cancer Panel issued their annual report revealing a link between exposure to synthetic pesticides and an increased number of cancer cases in farmworkers, as well as leukemia in children living in farming communities.[25] If this is what happens on the farm, what are these chemicals doing to our bodies when we eat them in small amounts day after day?

Food Babe Truth Detector:
The "Dose Makes the Poison" Fib

Critics say the amount of pesticides on food is too small to do any damage, but this isn't the case when talking about some of these chemicals, which are endocrine disruptors. According to the President's Cancer Panel: "The entire U.S. population is exposed on a daily basis to numerous agricultural chemicals, some of which also are used in residential and commercial landscaping. Many of these chemicals have known or suspected carcinogenic or endocrine disrupting properties. Pesticides (insecticides, herbicides, and fungicides) approved for use by the U.S. Environmental Protection Agency (EPA) contain nearly 900 active ingredients, many of which are toxic."[26]

Endocrine disruptors are substances that disrupt hormones and lead to reproductive problems, early onset puberty, obesity, diabetes, and some cancers. They are prevalent in our environment—we can't totally escape them. We come into constant contact with them on a daily basis through dietary and environmental exposure. When it comes to endocrine disruptors, it's been shown that chronic small exposures are damaging: "the dose makes the poison" mantra simply does not apply.[27]

WHAT ABOUT JUST PEELING AND WASHING THE PESTICIDES OFF?

It's not that easy. Many of the chemicals used on conventional food are systemic: meaning they're absorbed into the food and you can't simply just wash them off. There are often multiple pesticides in each fruit or vegetable—residue rates are rising, in fact—and there's no legal limit on the number of different pesticides found in food. When it comes to nonorganic packaged foods, you obviously cannot wash those. That's why so many of those processed snack foods that we discussed in the last chapter tested positive for glyphosate residues.

IT'S A MYTH THAT WE NEED PESTICIDES TO FEED THE WORLD

Big Food and Big Ag claim pesticides are needed to help "feed the world." But this is deceptive, since these very chemicals are badly damaging the environment. Experts at the U.N. recently warned that pesticides end up in our water systems, damage our ecological system, contaminate soils, are responsible for bee deaths, and are a huge environmental threat to the future of food production.[28] The issue of world hunger is due to poverty, inequality, and distribution—not lack of food.

"It's time to overturn the myth that pesticides are necessary to feed the world and create a global process to transition toward safer and healthier food and agricultural production," stated the U.N. Special Rapporteurs on Toxics and the Right to Food in March 2017.[29]

Certified Organic Label Lingo

What constitutes "organic"? Here's what all those labels actually mean.

- **100% organic.** Products are able to make this claim only if they are made with all organic ingredients (excluding water and salt). They may also put the USDA Organic seal on their packages.

- **Organic.** Products can also use the USDA Organic seal if they contain at least 95 percent organic ingredients (excluding water and salt). The remaining 5 percent cannot contain substances banned from organic foods, such as GMOs or artificial dyes.

- **Made with organic ingredients.** When you see this on a package, it contains at least 70 percent organic ingredients. These products are not permitted to use the USDA Organic seal.

Source: USDA Organic Labeling Standards[30]

ORGANIC PESTICIDES

Many consumers are confused about whether organic food production can ever involve pesticide and fertilizer use. Yes, they can—but with important distinctions. Organic farmers can apply organic certified pesticides and fungicides to their crops, as outlined and approved by the USDA Certified Organic program. They can also fertilize their crops with livestock manure. Before you turn up your nose, that's quite different from the sewage sludge (human waste) allowed in conventional farming. Scientific analysis has found that sewage sludge (aka "biosolids") is full of nasty bacteria, pharmaceuticals, toxic heavy metals, flame retardants, and other hazardous chemicals. (Now you can turn up your nose.) It's been shown that some of these contaminants are absorbed into (or remain as residue on) the crops we eat. Organic standards prohibit the use of this practice.[31]

Organic-approved pesticides are only allowed to be used as a "last resort" on organic crops after other methods fail, such as planting cover crops and mechanical weeding. Furthermore, farmers have to demonstrate the need for the pesticide to their organic certifier. In general, organic farmers are reluctant to use pesticides. When organic farmers do use them, they generally use natural and nontoxic substances derived from plants or bacteria.

Before a pesticide can even be approved for organics, it goes through many hoops and is more rigorously reviewed than other pesticides. That's why there are only about 25 synthetic products permitted on organic farms, while nonorganic farms have upward of 900 agrochemicals at their disposal.

These rules aren't perfect, but they help explain why tested organic produce contains much lower pesticide residues than nonorganic conventional produce.

Food Babe Truth Detector:
The Rotenone and Copper Sulfate Fibs

Critics argue that horribly toxic pesticides are used on organic crops, and that they're used in much greater amounts. Untrue. One of the pesticides they routinely bring up is rotenone, but this pesticide isn't even used in America. It was once approved for organic crops, but the EPA has banned it from U.S. crops (it's only registered for use as fish kill). Some other countries still use rotenone, and those crops may be imported as organic into the U.S., but the National Organic Standards Board has passed a recommendation to prohibit it outright.

Another one critics mention is copper sulfate. This can be used by both organic and conventional fruit farmers as a fungicide, but conventional farmers reportedly use more of it and their versions contain riskier "non-active" ingredients. Organic farmers are required to monitor copper sulfate use and aren't permitted to continue using the chemical if it accumulates in high levels in the soil.

Why Organic Meat Is Worth the Cost

If you eat meat or dairy, choosing organic is even more important. Conventional meat, eggs, and dairy can be contaminated with even more synthetic pesticides than plant-based foods. Pesticides used on feed accumulate in animal tissues over time, and pesticide residues have been found in conventional beef, egg, milk, pork, and poultry samples.[32] Using only Certified Organic feed is a requirement when raising organic animals.

Most conventional animals are also raised on growth-promoting steroids, antibiotics, and other drugs, and these residues have been found in meat.[33] The overuse of growth-promoting antibiotics is creating superbugs that contaminate the meat, putting us at greater risk of antibiotic-resistant infections. These drugs are prohibited in the raising of organic animals.

ACTION STEPS: GO ORGANIC

Buy USDA certified 100 percent organic food.

Any food claiming it is organic and that has the USDA Organic label on it is not allowed to have GMOs in any of the ingredients.

Be careful when choosing animal foods, too, since a majority of livestock in the U.S. are fed GMO grains, or are treated with the GMO bovine growth hormone rBGH—another Monsanto product. Do you really want to drink "Monsanto Milk" or eat "Monsanto Butter" derived from animals that have been fed GMO corn and soy heavily sprayed with harmful weed killers?

Make food choices to avoid pesticides.

We definitely need to eat more fruits and vegetables. The evidence is strong and overwhelming that they help protect against heart disease and cancer, ensure a healthy microbiome, and allow us to maintain a healthy weight. So keep produce front and center on your plate. I realize, of course, that some organic fruits and veggies can be rather expensive and are not always available, so if you can't go 100 percent organic, I suggest sticking with those fruits and veggies that generally have the least pesticide residue. Here's information from the Environmental Working Group that will help you make the best choices.

The Dirty Dozen

Make these foods a priority on your organic shopping list because conventional versions of these foods have been found to have the most pesticide residues:

1. Strawberries
2. Spinach
3. Nectarines
4. Apples
5. Grapes
6. Peaches
7. Cherries
8. Pears
9. Tomatoes
10. Celery
11. Potatoes
12. Sweet Bell Peppers

The Clean 15

The following foods, organic or not, are least likely to contain pesticide residues:

1. Avocados
2. * Sweet Corn
3. Pineapples
4. Cabbage
5. Onions
6. Sweet peas, frozen
7. * Papayas
8. Asparagus
9. Mangoes
10. Eggplants
11. Honeydew melons
12. Kiwis
13. Cantaloupes
14. Cauliflower
15. Broccoli

* A small amount of fresh sweet corn, papaya, and summer squash sold in the United States is produced from genetically modified seeds. Buy organic varieties of these crops if you want to avoid genetically modified produce.
Source: 2018 Shopper's Guide to Pesticides in Produce by the Environmental Working Group, ewg.org[34]

CHEMICAL FREE IS THE WAY TO BE

Next time you hear that organic food is a scam, remember which companies are paying for that message. They have a vested interest in convincing you that pesticides and herbicides are harmless. The evidence suggests otherwise.

Ultimately, the only person you can trust is yourself. Going organic is a personal choice, and with sales of organic foods increasing about 10 percent each year for the past decade, it's also an increasingly popular choice. Make the switch to organic food and see how you feel.

I think you'll be pleasantly surprised. Some things are worth paying extra for.

CHAPTER 12

Three Questions That Will Transform Your Health

When I was a kid, I was always asking questions. I'm happy to report that my inquisitive nature never left me. In high school, I became a nationally ranked debater and was recruited to the top debate colleges around the country. After I became a food activist, I dug deep into the skills I learned as a debater and started researching the most nutritious and healing foods on the planet. I also decided to figure out what was in the food I had been eating. I investigated food issues ferociously, because my own health issues had shown me the importance of the subject. I discovered the ugly truth behind additives, that food coloring is made from petrochemicals and the bodies of ground-up insects, why preservatives can cause cancer, how the sugar and flavor industries create addictive foods, and so much more.

I believe it's imperative that we eat the healthiest food possible. Good nutrition is about feeling better, looking better, and living longer. But with guilty parties lying to us about the food they sell, it gets harder all the time to sort the useful advice from the flawed or false.

I have a solution: become your own food investigator. Educate yourself about what you're buying in the grocery store and putting on your plate. Learning about what you eat fosters both the desire to live well and the confidence to weigh conflicting advice from different parties.

This is easier than you think. You don't have to make a full-time career of food activism and investigating like I have. You just need to ask, and answer, three simple questions about food:

1. What are the ingredients?
2. Are these ingredients nutritious?
3. Where do these ingredients come from?

Write these questions down and tuck a note in your wallet or purse. Hang them on your fridge. Save them in the notes in your phone. That's really all there is to it. I believe that if you can select food based on your answers to these three questions, you'll put yourself—and your loved ones—on the path to a healthy lifestyle right away. Plus, you'll be fighting back against those guilty parties who are trying to contaminate our foods in the name of profits.

Head into your kitchen right now and give these three questions a try. Yes, really right now. Go ahead and open up your fridge or pantry and grab one of your favorite food items. Now let's take a closer look.

QUESTION #1: WHAT ARE THE INGREDIENTS?

This is probably the most important of the three questions. Know what is in your food. For starters, you must read ingredient labels. If the food contains any additives or preservatives, ask yourself why they are used and whether they're really necessary.

If you don't know what an ingredient or additive is or how it can affect your health, put the product back and look for a product made with real food instead.

The front of the package tells you very little about what's really in a product. This is the primary place where most consumers look when choosing healthy products, but this is a big mistake! Food manufacturers know this, and exploit it to their advantage. Take a bottle of V8 Splash Fruit Medley juice drink, for instance. The front label has brightly colored pictures of fruit and boldly claims it contains antioxidant vitamins A and C, which certainly gives the impression that it's a healthy food. However, the ingredients list paints another story, as you'll find its first two ingredients are water and high-fructose corn syrup—making these the most prominent ingredients in this drink. As you read down the ingredients list, you'll further find that it's artificially colored with Red #40 (made from petroleum) and sweetened up even more with the artificial sweetener sucralose (made by chlorinating sugar molecules). V8 Splash may contain those antioxidants A and C, but you'll be gulping them down with copious amounts of sugar and chemical additives. Now that doesn't seem very healthy, does it?

There's an erroneous implication out there that all the ingredients allowed in processed food—preservatives, artificial sweeteners, thickeners, stabilizers, emulsifiers—have gone through some sort of rigorous safety testing by the FDA proving they're okay to eat, but in many cases they haven't. As we discussed in Chapter 3, new ingredients are often approved by the food manufacturers themselves, and not by the FDA, and it's a system fraught with loopholes. This is why we need to take responsibility for our own health and not rely on the FDA (or anyone else) to protect us from all the additives and untested chemicals in our food.

The bottom line: try to stick to whole foods with simple ingredients lists. The fewer unnecessary ingredients added to your food, the better. The more real whole foods you eat, the healthier your body will be. Examples: fresh fruits, fresh vegetables, nuts and seeds, legumes, and lean meats—all organic if possible. Choosing real food is the simplest way to answer this question without having any doubts.

QUESTION #2: ARE THESE INGREDIENTS NUTRITIOUS?

It makes me incredibly sad that people out there are doing whatever it takes to get healthy and look and feel their best—but are facing an uphill battle because of what the food industry has done to our food and the way they are marketing it to us.

Marketing terms like "diet," "light," "free," "natural," and "healthy" are blazoned on food packages that are filled with controversial additives that provide the body with zero nutrition. What kind of viable nutrition does your body get when you nosh on Yellow #5, carrageenan, and natural flavors? The answer is none.

When it comes to the additives in our food, it makes sense to be wary. The majority of food additives invented in the last few decades have been created with the sole purpose of improving the bottom line of the food industry, not with our health or nutrition in mind.

This is why it is so important to look critically at our food choices. Thus, an easy way to answer this question is to clarify whether the food is "whole" or "processed." A food that is "whole" simply means a food as found in nature. Whole foods are typically "one-ingredient foods" and they don't contain any preservatives, dyes, or any of the additives listed in the Appendix.

Whole food is real food: real meat, real broccoli, real apples. If the food and its ingredients don't fit the descriptions of whole and real, chances are they're not good for you. Eating a well-balanced diet packed with whole, fresh foods is vital to health, energy, and longevity.

Rather than a food sweetened with sugar (which is highly refined and devoid of nutrients), it's better to choose one sweetened with dates, maple syrup, or honey (which all contain healthy nutrients from nature). Instead of a food made with bleached wheat flour that is "enriched" with synthetic vitamins and minerals, choose those made with whole organic grains, nuts, seeds, and other healthy foods.

The first thing many people look for on a product is the calorie count because they believe the lie that it really doesn't matter where your calories come from, as long as you don't eat too many of them. This theory is broken and leads people down the path of eating heavily processed foods full of artificial sweeteners, thickeners, and other health-wrecking additives that are devoid of nutrients. Instead, start focusing on whether a food is nutritious or not. That's the key question. Instead of focusing on the quantity of calories, fat grams, or carbs we eat, it's more important to emphasize the *quality* of those calories. Seek out nutrition first and the rest will follow.

Avoid Processed Foods to Cut Cancer Risk

One recent study by European scientists in the prestigious *British Medical Journal* carefully tracked the diets of more than 100,000 participants. Then they looked at how different diets influenced the likelihood of getting cancer. Their main finding was that people who ate more "ultraprocessed foods"—think mass-produced breads, cookies, chicken nuggets, sodas, instant soups, junk like that—were more likely to get cancer. The numbers are telling: a 10 percent increase in ultraprocessed foods led to a 12 percent increase in cancer incidence.[1]

While the researchers note that this correlation between junk food and cancer could be caused by many factors—there's so much wrong with ultraprocessed food, it's hard to know where to start—suspected culprits include food packaging materials and the cocktail of additives in these foods with the potential to create interactions in our bodies.

QUESTION #3: WHERE DO THESE INGREDIENTS COME FROM?

When you shop for food, or dine out, you deserve to know where that food comes from, and people overwhelmingly tell me they *want* to know. Unless you do all your shopping at a local farmers market, the produce you buy has generally made a journey from grower to packer to distributor to supplier to grocery store. Preservatives were probably used to extend shelf life, or the food was cultivated with pesticides, chemicals, fertilizer, antibiotics, and growth hormones.

Still, there are ways you can trace your food back to its source. Look at its PLU (price look-up) number. A 9 at the beginning of a five-digit sequence indicates the produce is organically grown. A four-digit code beginning with a 3 or 4 means it was conventionally grown and may be GMO if it's a GMO crop. The current list of GMO crops includes corn, potatoes, apples, zucchini, yellow squash, and papaya. You can also use apps like HarvestMark for more tracing.

As for animal proteins, it's best to avoid meat from animals raised on conventional factory farms (which are notorious for using hormones and other growth-promoting drugs, while feeding the animals antibiotics and GMO feed in cramped and unsanitary conditions). The vast majority of meat in the average grocery store is from these types of farms, even if it's labeled "all natural." The best strategy is to look for labels that really mean something, such as Animal Welfare Approved, Certified Humane, and Certified Organic.

When I eat meat, I always try to buy local and organic. One of the best ways to obtain meat and other foods that are optimum for your health is to buy directly from local farms, where you can shake the farmer's hand and talk with them. You can connect online with farmers markets or use subscription-based Community Supported Agriculture (CSAs) to purchase organic meat that wasn't raised in a cramped and filthy factory farm.

Buying animal products directly from the farmer is becoming increasingly common. I like to know that food animals had a "free-range" life and weren't kept in a crate and pumped with antibiotics in some Big Ag operation. Ideally, my meat comes from a healthy, contented cow that grazed on an open, green pasture its whole life.

And it's not just meat: I try to buy as much food as possible directly from my local farmers. Eating locally puts you in touch with the person who produced what you're about to eat. This way you support local agriculture, and enjoy food that is more nutrient dense because it hasn't been preserved to travel hundreds of miles to your store. If you'd like to learn how to do so, you can connect online with farmers markets, subscription-based CSAs, buying clubs, and farms at:

- LocalHarvest.org
- EatWild.com

At restaurants, when a plate of food is placed before you, have you ever thought about where it has come from and how it was prepared?

It's easy to order and just eat . . . right?

Yes, it's easy . . . but it's just as easy to ask where your meal comes from. Some tips: ***Quiz the restaurant about its meat supplier.*** When you're dining out, ask your server where the restaurant purchases its meat. If they don't know, or say it's dropped off by Sysco or some other huge distributor, that indicates the meat is probably processed to the hilt. Don't eat the meat or dairy at a restaurant unless you know it's raised without antibiotics.

The same goes for fish: make sure it's wild caught and not farm raised.

Find out which cooking fats are used. Restaurants are notorious for frying food in unhealthy inflammatory oils like "soybean oil" or "vegetable oil." Check with the kitchen before ordering and ask what type of cooking oil they use. Go so far as to ask them to read the actual ingredients list on the oil container.

Learn whether the restaurant uses GMO food. When you go out to eat, ask your server if the food is non-GMO. He or she might not know, but at least you'll start educating your favorite restaurants and their workers. If an item isn't organic and contains a common GMO crop (like corn), choose other items instead that are not at risk of being GMO.

Lean toward homemade. Before you order soup or other dishes at a restaurant, ask if it's homemade or if it contains additives.

Order something not on the menu. Ask the chef to create something for you. This request can be made easily at a fancier or more established restaurant where chefs are highly skilled and can experiment for you. Ask for your meat to be simply prepared with olive oil or butter and salt, or ask for steamed fresh vegetables.

Build a relationship with a favorite restaurant. When I'm too busy to cook but still want to eat healthy, I head to my favorite standby. I've gotten to know the staff and they make everything perfect for me every time. For example, my favorite sushi chef prepares a special roll with all veggies and no white rice or unhealthy sauces. He calls it the "Food Babe Roll." He also knows that I like my ponzu sauce on the side of my sashimi. I always start with a big bowl of romaine with extra cucumbers and the ginger dressing on the side, and they serve great hot green tea. My meals there are fail-proof, and I never have to stress about what I'm eating.

Look, I know it's hard to insist on eating right when you eat out, especially when you're dining with a group. When I first started asking questions at restaurants, people teased me. "Oh, Vani is about to order. Time to take a nap!" Or, "The restaurant is going to hate us. Vani is ordering!" But after I left the hospital, I promised myself I'd stick to my principles. And sometimes, people even came to appreciate it.

There was one time I was invited to dinner at a fancy steakhouse. After looking at the menu and asking questions about the meat, I realized that I didn't want anything on the menu. So I asked the chef if he could make me a vegetable plate instead. I was pretty nervous to do that if front of all the people I was with, so I whispered my order to the waiter. However, when the food came out, my vegetarian meal looked so much better that they started asking if they could get the same thing.

We all want to eat food that makes us feel good. Sometimes, we just need to be reminded that we can: it only requires that we read the ingredients and investigate what's really in all those packaged and processed items. Because it's time to stop outsourcing our food decisions to Big Food. It's time to stop feeling awful. It's time to stop getting sick and gaining weight. It's time to take back control of our food supply from these companies that just want our money and don't give a damn about health.

Of course, starting the food revolution we need won't be easy, and it won't happen overnight. I have no doubt that food companies will do everything possible to keep feeding us their highly lucrative junk food. But none of us needs to succumb to industry lies and ties. The truth is out there. If all we did was stop eating processed food and instead build our diet around whole, organic, and real food, we'd shield ourselves automatically from most chemicals, toxins, added sugar, and other additives in food.

Nobody's perfect. We all have days when we end up eating something that we know isn't good for us. That's why it's important to remember that making major lifestyle changes—and changing how you eat is one of the biggest changes you can make—is an ever-evolving process that involves recognizing what will and will not work for you. My goal is to simply keep you informed and help you see through the industry-funded lies so you can choose the best foods for yourself. Big Food spends hundreds of millions of dollars every year persuading us that it's okay to drink toxic sodas and eat foods made out of chemicals we can't pronounce. And then, when we get sick, they invest in propaganda that tells us it's just our fault for not exercising enough. It's time to stop believing them. It's time to take back control.

Knowledge is power.

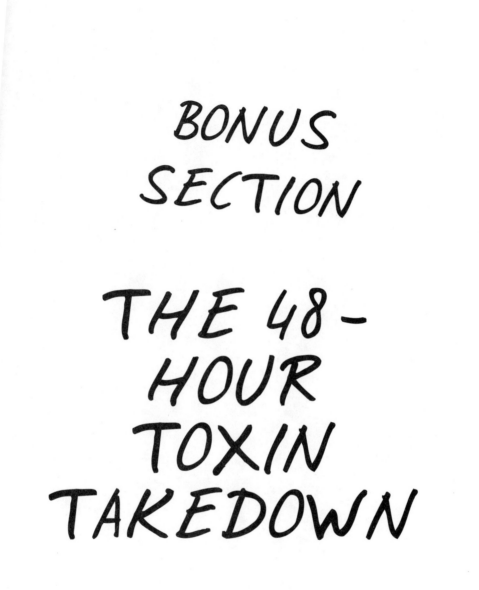

BONUS SECTION

THE 48-HOUR TOXIN TAKEDOWN

The 48-Hour
Toxin Takedown
Plan

What we eat is the single most important factor shaping how we feel. In part, this is because our diet determines how well we defend ourselves from exposure to toxins, both in the environment and in our food. We can accumulate those toxins by ingesting or inhaling chemicals from household cleaners, beauty products, air pollution, pesticides, heavy metals, and even additives in our food. We also know that eating foods loaded with salt, sugar, denatured fats, or just too many calories can harm our health, leading to a number of chronic diseases, including heart disease and diabetes.

The result of exposure can be the gradual accumulation of toxins in your body that, in turn, can put a major burden on your body's organs of elimination. The liver, kidneys, skin, and intestines, which normally filter out wastes and toxins, can become overloaded and have difficulty doing their jobs.

When this happens, your digestion, circulation, and metabolism can be thrown out of whack. You may experience symptoms such as constipation, bloating, weight gain, poor skin tone, and fatigue—and vulnerability to chronic health problems if toxic exposure goes unchecked.

In addition to helping us avoid harmful health effects and improve our well-being, certain foods help our bodies detoxify from health-injuring substances. They do this by boosting the action of "detoxification enzymes," which help filter the blood and eliminate toxins. Science already tells us, for example, that people who eat a lot of brassica vegetables, such as broccoli, cabbage, and cauliflower, tend to have a lower lifetime risk of getting cancer.[1] One of the reasons is that these veggies contain an anti-cancer chemical called indole-3-carbinol.[2] It maximizes the work of detoxification enzymes in the liver, which in turn helps prevent the buildup of carcinogens in the body.

Produced naturally in the body, detoxification enzymes are found in every organ system in the body, including the breast, lung, stomach, and liver. These enzymes are your first line of defense against all the toxins that come into your body. This is why the food you eat is so important: it ramps up their power.

So I believe in "detox" diets, provided they focus on whole foods that are rich in the right kind of detoxification enzymes. My 48-Hour Toxin Takedown is a two-day plan in which you'll infuse your body with a high concentration of foods that boost the action of these enzymes and help your body maximize its ability to purge itself of environmental toxins. Later on, and hopefully for a lifetime, you'll incorporate these foods and nutrients into your diet so that your detoxification enzymes can do their work, day in and day out, and rid your system of unwanted toxins.

I understand that the thought of detoxing for a week, 10 days, or more can be daunting—which is why I've made it easy for you with this simple, delicious 48-hour plan. You don't need to drastically transform your lifestyle to detox and feel better. All you need is 48 hours.

Research backs me up on this. An excellent example has to do with BPA (bisphenol A), a toxic chemical used to line canned foods and soft drinks. As an endocrine disruptor, it messes with your hormones and can lead to cancer, obesity, and reproductive issues.

A 2012 study conducted by researchers at the EPA found that a 48-hour fast of drinking water eliminated significant amounts of BPA in people who had this chemical in their systems.[3] I'm definitely not advocating a two-day water fast, but this study shows that a nasty toxin like BPA can leave the body rather quickly, given the right resources. You can certainly give your body some extra vitality with a short detox plan like this one.

SHOULD YOU DO THE 48-HOUR TOXIN TAKEDOWN?

You may or may not need this plan, so let's get personal for a moment. Like any machine, the body won't run smoothly if it's overburdened and poorly maintained. What would cause that to happen? An overindulgent weekend or vacation isn't the sole culprit—it's more to do with our daily dietary habits. Even those who keep fit and try to eat a balanced diet should look closely at what they eat. Does your diet include a lot of take-out food, convenience and refined foods, or alcohol? Do you skip meals, sometimes overeat, have late nights, and drink lots of coffee the next day to recharge? Do you have a lot of stress? Do you live in a polluted area? If you do one or more of these things, you may be taking in more toxins than you realize. The Toxin Takedown will be a good introduction to detoxing.

THE BENEFITS

By giving your body certain foods and nutrients for 48 hours, you're fortifying your detoxification system and allowing your body to detox on its own.

- The plan itself will probably help zap cravings for your usual sugary, fatty snacks.
- Your skin and hair may improve, even after only two days.
- You may experience improved energy levels, digestion, and brain activity.

WAYS TO USE THE 48-HOUR TOXIN TAKEDOWN

You can try this for 48 hours to see how you feel and continue on from there by following a consistently healthy, organic diet with foods that support detoxification.

Or you can use the Takedown as a form of "intermittent fasting"—in other words, use it once a week. An intermittent fast has been shown in research to be one of the most effective interventions for normalizing your weight, activating your body's fat-burning mode, regulating blood sugar, reducing your risk of chronic disease, and preventing dementia.[4]

Another way to incorporate the Takedown is for "damage control": say, after a weekend when you've overindulged on alcohol, sweets, too much sodium, processed foods, and so forth.

You can even extend the Takedown to five or seven days, if you're brave and like your results. A 2000 study published in *Alternative Therapies in Health and Medicine* investigated whether a seven-day detox was beneficial. The diet included fruits, vegetables, nuts and seeds, rice, legumes, and optional foods, such as turkey, fish, and various grains (buckwheat, millet, amaranth, quinoa, and brown rice). Not allowed were sweets, caffeine products, alcohol, eggs, or gluten-containing foods. In many ways, the food plan was similar to the 48-Hour Toxin Takedown. After the seven-day experimental period ended, all laboratory measures showed improved detoxification capacity, and the participants reported that they felt better.[5]

But whenever you use it, the 48-Hour Toxin Takedown is for two days only. You can do it.

WHAT TO EAT FOR THE NEXT 48 HOURS

Many detox diets advise that you eat or drink very little, but those are tough recommendations to follow. Furthermore, they don't really support your detoxification enzyme processes. My plan is both more realistic and scientific. It focuses on foods that are filled with vitamins, antioxidants, fiber, and nutrients that the body requires for detoxification. This plan focuses on clean eating in which you eat whole, organic foods rather than processed ones. These foods include vegetables, fruits, whole grains, and lean protein. It fully minimizes the amount of chemical intake and focuses only on eating organic foods. For two days, you will reward your body with wholesome foods and rid your system of waste and toxins. You can eat:

VEGETABLES

I don't believe anyone would dispute that vegetables are superior for health. Huge amounts of scientific evidence prove that the more vegetables you eat, the lower your risk of chronic diseases—for at least three vital reasons. First, vegetables are an abundant source of vitamins and minerals. Second, the antioxidants and phytochemicals they contain, in particular, activate detoxification enzymes. Third, these foods stimulate your immune system, prevent abnormal blood clotting, reduce blood pressure, and generally protect against chronic diseases.

The Takedown focuses on some key detoxification foods:

Artichokes. Few detoxifying diets would be complete without artichokes, which taste delicious on salads. It's been shown that artichoke leaves have properties that stimulate production of bile, which helps shuttle toxins out of your liver, and ultimately, out of your body.[6] Artichokes are also packed with the antioxidants, including silymarin (known to protect the liver from toxins).

Beans. You can substitute ¾ cup of black beans for animal protein on the Takedown, as well as put them on salads. Beans are a top source of fiber, which scrubs your digestive tract so that it's free of toxins. They also provide the protein from which phase I and phase II enzymes are manufactured.

Beets. This often underrated but highly nutritious veggie has been the subject of many research studies that have shown its health benefits. Beets contain an antioxidant called betanin, which increases the activity of phase II detoxification enzymes, according to a 2013 study published in the *British Journal of*

Nutrition.[7] The researchers found that betanin protects the liver—the body's main organ of detoxification—and helps prevent cancer.

Brassica vegetables. These include kale, broccoli, brussels sprouts, cauliflower, and cabbage. These are excellent sources of phytochemicals known to turn on our detoxification enzymes and protect against cancer.

Cilantro. This popular salsa ingredient has a direct "chelating" (removal) effect on a number of heavy metals including mercury and lead, both of which are highly toxic to the body, particularly the brain.

Garlic and onions. Sure, you have to have a lot of mouthwash on hand if you eat a lot of garlic and onions, but enjoying these veggies on a regular basis powerfully boosts the activity of phase 2 detoxification enzymes, according to a *Free Radical Biology and Medicine* report published in 2003.[8]

Green leafy vegetables. Spinach, kale, collards, lettuces, and other green leafy vegetables are thought to be responsible for several beneficial properties such as antioxidant, anti-cancer, and detoxification activities, according to a study in *PeerJ* published in 2016.[9] The report mentions that one of the key detoxifying components in these veggies is chlorophyll, which gives these foods their green color. This pigment helps plants absorb light energy for use in photosynthesis and growth, and it is essential to all life on earth.

Probiotic/fermented vegetables. Two fermented foods are included in the plan: kimchi and sauerkraut. Kimchi is a traditional fermented Korean side dish made of vegetables with a variety of seasonings. It is teeming with probiotics. The major ingredients of kimchi are brassica vegetables, along with other detox foods and spices, including garlic, ginger, and red pepper powder. A 2014 review of kimchi published in the *Journal of Medicinal Food* listed its numerous health benefits.[10] Kimchi fights obesity, constipation and other digestive problems, abnormally high cholesterol levels, immune disorders, poor skin, and brain degeneration. No wonder kimchi is my favorite fermented food.

As for sauerkraut, it is just as powerful a detox food. Not only does it supply probiotics, but it is made solely from cabbage. Cabbage contains compounds known as glucosinolates, which turn on our detoxification enzymes and help the liver, according to an article published in *The Journal of Nutrition* in 2005, along with many other studies found in the scientific literature.[11]

FRUIT

You'll enjoy two fresh fruits daily (and some fruit as a part of fresh-made juice). The fruits I recommend for detoxification are any of the citrus fruits—such as oranges, lemons, and grapefruit—and berries. Citrus fruits contain limonoids, which influence the activity of phase II detoxifying enzymes, according to a study in *BMC Complementary and Alternative Medicine* in 2010.[12] Berries, such as blueberries, raspberries, strawberries, blackberries, and cranberries, do the trick too. They are loaded with flavonoids, natural plant nutrients that increase the activity of liver detoxification enzymes.

Fruits (and veggies) are also a good source of soluble and insoluble fiber, which help usher toxins out of the intestinal tract. Fruits in general are also high in water content, which aids in detoxification.

GRAINS

These foods are "absorbent" carbohydrates, meaning that they're brilliant for clutching on to and clearing out toxic waste buildup in the intestines. The two grains I emphasize on this plan are quinoa and steel cut oats.

Although technically not a grain (it is referred to as a grain because it resembles grains in appearance), quinoa is actually a seed. The kernels can be red, black, white, or golden in color. It does not contain gluten, making it a terrific carb if you're sensitive to gluten in any way, and it does not belong to the same plant family as wheat. It's an excellent source of B vitamins, potassium, and phytonutrients.

I like the choice of steel cut oats, for three reasons: They taste delicious. They retain more nutrients than rolled oats and other varieties. And they're packed with detoxifying fiber.

LEAN PROTEINS

You have the choice of organic free-range chicken or wild-caught salmon for dinner. (Vegetarians and vegan can opt for black beans or lentils.) All are high-quality, well-absorbed proteins that supply key amino acids that help manufacture detox-ification enzymes in the body.

FATS AND OILS

I recommend coconut oil for detoxification, mainly because it provides quick carb-like fuel for energy. Coconut oil is made up primarily of medium-chain triglycerides (MCTs), a type of fat that is metabolized differently from other fats. It is less likely to be stored as fat and has a thermogenic effect, meaning that it increases fat burning. It also has antimicrobial properties and helps restore gut health.

Another terrific food fat is avocado. Besides supplying essential fats for whole-body health, the avocado is a significant source of glutathione, an important detoxifying substance in the liver.

DAIRY

The Takedown includes grass or pastured-raised dairy yogurt. Yogurt provides probiotics for gut health and intestinal detoxification. Because it contains protein, yogurt provides amino acids necessary for creating phase II detoxifying enzymes.

SEEDS

Pumpkin seeds and flaxseeds are included on the plan. Pumpkin seeds pack a punch in terms of protein, healthy fats, carotenoids, and vitamin E. In research, they've been found to help control blood sugar, fight cancer, normalize blood pressure, and protect the heart.[13] A source of good fats, flaxseeds are excellent for "spring cleaning" the intestinal tract to eliminate toxins.

BOTH DAYS FOR THE NEXT 48 HOURS—GUIDELINES

- Eat whole, organic foods. This will limit the amount of food additives and toxins you ingest from processed foods, making it easier for your liver to do its job.

- Each day, drink at least 64 ounces of spring or filtered water to help flush out toxins. This also helps your body absorb nutrients.

- Include herbal teas in addition to water. Good choices include decaffeinated green tea, dandelion, hibiscus, chamomile (best in the evening because this herb promotes restful sleep), mint, and dandelion.

- Drink a cup of warm lemon water with cayenne pepper as soon as you get up in the morning. Squeeze one-half of the lemon into a cup of warm water, and sprinkle with cayenne pepper (for extra detoxifying and metabolism boosting). If you don't like lemon or cayenne, lime water or apple cider vinegar is a great substitute.

- For midmorning and midafternoon snacks, enjoy a glass of my *48-Hour Toxin Takedown Juice* (page 223), made with vegetables known to rid the body of toxins. The juice recipe also calls for the addition of super green powder, a supplement that contains spirulina, chlorella, wheatgrass, and other concentrated plant sources of detoxifying nutrients.

- What you'll have to give up for 48 hours: coffee, caffeinated foods, regular tea, salt, dairy products (with the exception of yogurt), alcohol, sweets, sweeteners (including artificial sweeteners), soft drinks, diet drinks, nondairy coffee creamers, and any processed foods.

THE PLAN

Day 1:

First thing in the morning: warm lemon juice.

Breakfast: 1 to 2 pieces of organic fruit and 2 table-spoons of ground flaxseed mixed with pasture-raised dairy yogurt or steel cut oats.

Midmorning: *Takedown Juice.*

Lunch: Large salad of raw greens (baby spinach, baby kale, arugula) topped with other veggies such as artichokes, broccoli florets, shredded carrots, red onion, sliced hard-boiled egg (optional), and raw pumpkin seeds. Drizzle with *Coconut Oil Dressing.*

Midafternoon: *Takedown Juice.*

Dinner: *Quinoa Stir-Fry.* Option to add lentils, black beans, chicken or fish.

Day 2:

First thing in the morning: warm lemon juice.

Breakfast: 1 to 2 pieces of organic fruit and 2 table-spoons of ground flaxseed mixed with pastured-raised dairy yogurt or steel cut oats.

Midmorning: *Takedown Juice.*

Lunch: *Simple Avocado Salad* with artichoke hearts, drizzled with *Coconut Oil Dressing*, served on sliced organic tomato; or green raw salad from Day 1; or left-over *Quinoa Stir-Fry* (as a time saver).

Midafternoon: *Takedown Juice.*

Dinner: Grilled wild salmon or grilled chicken breast or 3/4 cup black beans or lentils; *Garlic Mashed Cauliflower*; small mixed green salad with balsamic vinegar; and side of kimchi or sauerkraut.

Shopping List for the 48-Hour Toxin Takedown

Organic Vegetables (produce section):

- Small packages of baby kale, baby spinach, arugula, dandelion greens, and lettuce
- Tomato, 1 medium
- Red onion, 1 small
- Shredded carrots, one small bag
- Carrot, 1 whole
- Beets, 1 to 2
- Avocado, 1
- Cauliflower, 1 small head
- Garlic, 1 bulb
- Broccoli florets
- Cilantro, 1 bunch
- Parsley, 1 bunch
- Cucumbers, 2
- Red bell pepper, 1
- Bok choy, 1 bunch
- Scallions, 1 bunch
- Chives, 1 bunch
- Gingerroot, 1 small piece
- Turmeric root, 1 small piece (or ground turmeric)

Organic Fruits (produce section):

- Green apple, 1
- Organic fruit of your choosing for Day 1 and 2 breakfasts
- Lemon, 3
- Limes, 2

Canned Vegetables:

- Black beans, one 15-ounce can
- Dried lentils (2 cups)
- Chickpeas, one 15-ounce can
- Artichoke hearts, one 15-ounce can

Grains:

- Quinoa, one package
- Steel cut oats, one carton

Lean Proteins:

- Salmon fillet, 6 to 8 ounces
- Chicken breast, 6 to 8 ounces

Dairy:

- Pasture-raised yogurt, two 6-ounce cartons (if using)
- Grass-fed butter, one small package (if using)
- Eggs, small package (if using)

Other:

- Cayenne pepper, one jar
- Coconut oil, one small bottle
- Flaxseeds, one small packet

- Pumpkin seeds, one small packet
- Kimchi, one small carton, or one small jar of sauerkraut
- Balsamic vinegar, one small bottle
- Raw honey, one small jar
- Low sodium tamari, one small bottle
- Extra virgin olive oil, one small bottle

The 48-Hour Toxin Takedown Recipes

TAKEDOWN JUICE

Serves 1

Prep Time: 10 minutes

2 cups dandelion greens, kale, or spinach

1 cucumber

1 handful parsley

1-inch piece gingerroot

1 green apple, core removed

½ lemon, peel removed

Wash all vegetables thoroughly before juicing.

Juice each vegetable in this order: greens, cucumber, parsley, ginger, apple, and lemon. Stir before serving. Enjoy!

COCONUT OIL DRESSING

Serves 1

Prep Time: 5 minutes

2 tablespoons melted coconut oil

2 tablespoons lemon juice

1 clove garlic, peeled and minced

1 teaspoon raw honey

½ teaspoon grated turmeric root (or ¼ teaspoon ground turmeric)

Sea salt and ground pepper, to taste

Place all of the ingredients in a bowl and whisk vigorously to combine. Serve with your favorite salad. Enjoy!

QUINOA STIR-FRY

Serves 1

Prep Time: 10 minutes

Cook Time: 15 minutes

1 tablespoon coconut oil

1 teaspoon grated gingerroot

1 carrot, sliced on the bias

½ red bell pepper, sliced

½ cup chopped bok choy

1 scallion, chopped

2 tablespoons low sodium tamari

1 cup cooked quinoa

Sea salt and ground pepper, to taste

Heat the oil in a sauté pan over medium heat.

Add the ginger and cook for 1 minute. Add the carrot, pepper, bok choy, and scallion and cook for 4 to 5 minutes.

Add the tamari and 2 tablespoons of filtered water and cook for 2 to 3 minutes.

Add the quinoa to the sauté pan and mix to combine. Season with salt and pepper and serve. Enjoy!

SIMPLE AVOCADO SALAD

Serves 1

Prep Time: 10 minutes

1 avocado, peeled, pitted, and chopped

½ cup cooked chickpeas

½ small cucumber, diced

½ small red onion, sliced

2 tablespoons chopped cilantro

2 tablespoons extra virgin olive oil

2 tablespoons lime juice

Sea salt and pepper, to taste

Place all of the ingredients in a bowl and mix well to combine.

Serve over choice of greens or by itself. Enjoy!

GARLIC MASHED CAULIFLOWER

Serves 1

Prep Time: 10 minutes

Cook Time: 10 minutes

2 cups chopped cauliflower florets

1 clove garlic, peeled

1 teaspoon grass-fed butter

Sea salt and pepper, to taste

2 tablespoons chopped chives

Bring a pot of water to boil. Add the cauliflower and garlic clove and cook 8 to 10 minutes or until tender.

Drain thoroughly and place back in the pot. Add the butter and mash with a masher until a creamy puree has formed. Season with salt and pepper.

Stir in the chives and serve warm. Enjoy!

Lifelong Detox: Where to Go from Here

If you liked the feeling of detoxing for 48 hours and want to continue, there are daily food choices you can make to keep your body's detoxification system in peak condition. To lower your toxic burden, you can make "clean" choices most days of the week while avoiding problem foods that diminish your natural detoxification power.

Here is a list of foods, organized into food groups, that will help increase your body's ability to eliminate toxins:

DETOXIFYING FOOD CHOICES TO EAT DAILY AND WEEKLY		
Vegetables, Non-Starchy *Servings per day: Unlimited*		
Brassica Family		
Broccoflower	Cabbage	Kohlrabi
Broccoli	Cauliflower	Radishes
Detoxifying Leafy Greens		
Arugula	Endive	Spinach
Beet greens	Escarole	Swiss chard
Bok choy	Mustard greens	Turnip greens
Cilantro	Parsley	Watercress
Collard greens	Radicchio	
Dandelion greens	Romaine lettuce	
Detoxifying Boosters		
Garlic	Onion	Shallots
Leeks	Scallions	
Liver and Digestive Support		
Artichokes	Celery	
Asparagus	Sprouts, all types	
Other Cleansing Vegetables		
Carrots	Jicama	Squash
Cucumbers	Mushrooms	Tomatoes
Fennel	Peppers, all types	Turnips
Green beans	Sea vegetables	Vegetables, fermented

Vegetables, Starchy *Servings per day: 1*		
Beans or lentils, ½ cup	Hummus, ⅓ cup	Sweet potato, 1 medium
Beets, 1 cup	Parsnips, ½ cup	Winter squash (acorn, butternut squash), 1 cup
Corn, ½ cup	Peas, ½ cup	
Edamame, ½ cup	Rutabaga, ½ cup	

Fruits *Servings per day: 1*		
Apple, 1 medium	Grapes, ½ cup	Pear, 1 medium
Apricots, 2	Kiwi, 2	Pineapple, 1 cup
Banana, ½ medium	Mango, ½ small	Plum, 2
Blackberries, 1 cup	Melon, 1 cup	Raisins or dried cranberries, 2 tablespoons
Blueberries, 1 cup	Nectarine, 1 medium	Raspberries, 1 cup
Cherries, ½ cup	Orange, 1 medium	Strawberries, 1 cup
Dates, figs, or prunes, 3	Papaya, 1 cup	Tangerines, 2 small
Grapefruit, ½ fruit	Peach, 1 medium	

Grains, Cooked (Mostly Gluten Free)		
Amaranth, ½ cup	Oats, steel cut (not gluten free, but low in gluten)	
Buckwheat, ½ cup	Quinoa, ½ cup	Teff, ½ cup
Millet, ½ cup	Rice (basmati, black, brown, jasmine), ½ cup	

Lean Proteins *Servings per day: 2–3*		
Animal Protein		
I encourage grass-fed, pasture-raised, and free-range sources of animal protein because they are higher in healthy omega-3 fatty acids than their corn-fed and caged counterparts:		
Egg, 1	Fish, 4 to 6 ounces	Poultry, skinless, 4 to 6 ounces
Egg whites, 2	Low-fat meat, 4 to 6 ounces	
Plant Protein		
Beans and legumes (see above under Vegetables, Starchy)	Protein powder (hemp or pea) (1 scoop)	Tofu and tempeh (½ cup)

Fats and Oils *Servings per day: 1*	
Avocado, ½	Flaxseed oil, 1 tablespoon
Coconut oil, 1 tablespoon	Olive oil, 1 tablespoon

Dairy and Dairy Alternatives *Servings per day: 1*		
Kefir, 1 cup	Nondairy yogurts	Yogurt, 6 ounces
Nondairy milks (almond, cashew, coconut, hemp, rice, etc.), 1 cup		

Nuts and Seeds *Servings per day: 1 to 2*		
Almonds, 12	Hemp seeds, 1 tablespoon	Sesame seeds, 1 tablespoon
Brazil nuts, 2	Nut butter, 1 tablespoon	Sunflower seeds, 1 tablespoon
Cashews, 6	Pecans, 12	Teff, ½ cup
Chia seeds, 1 tablespoon	Pistachios, 16	Walnuts, 12
Flaxseeds, ground, 2 tablespoons	Pumpkin seeds, 1 tablespoon	

Appendix

Many packaged foods contain ingredients that can rob us of our health. As you read labels, become familiar with certain ingredients to avoid at all costs. Let's review them:

ACESULFAME POTASSIUM (ACE-K)

What it is: Artificial sweetener.

Why to avoid: The Center for Science in the Public Interest says to avoid it because safety testing done in the 1970s was inadequate.[1] See "Artificial Sweeteners."

Sources: Diet drinks, protein shakes and powders, fruit cups, yogurts, and "sugar-free" products.

ARTIFICIAL FLAVORS

What they are: Synthetic flavors made from proprietary chemicals.

Why to avoid: These are used to make fake food taste real and are a clear clue that the food you're eating is full of other bad things. Artificial flavors are not a single ingredient; each flavor may contain of up to 100 other ingredients, including synthetic chemicals, solvents, and preservatives such as BHA, propylene glycol, MSG, parabens, and more.

Sources: Cereal, candy, drink mixes, desserts, and soft drinks.

Artificial Sweeteners (In General)

What they are: Zero-calorie sweeteners such as aspartame and sucralose.

Why to avoid: Although they have no calories, artificial sweeteners have been shown to contribute to weight gain by encouraging sugar cravings.

Sources: Anything labeled "diet," "low calorie," "sugar free," or "reduced sugar."

Aspartame (NutraSweet)

What it is: Artificial sweetener.

Reasons to avoid: Studies show that artificial sweeteners encourage sugar craving and sugar dependence and are thereby linked to weight gain.[2] In addition, research has linked aspartame to various medical conditions, though more research is needed.[3]

Sources: Diet drinks, protein shakes and powders, fruit cups, yogurts, chewing gum, "sugar-free" products.

Azodicarbonamide (aka the "Yoga Mat Chemical")

What it is: Dough conditioner.

Reasons to avoid: The World Health Organization has linked it to respiratory issues, allergies, and asthma. When the azodicarbonamide in bread is baked, there is research that links it to tumor development and cancer. Semicarbazide (a carcinogen)[4] and urethane[5] (a suspected carcinogen) can form from azodicarbonamide during baking. This additive is banned in Europe and Australia, and the Center for Science in the Public Interest has called on the FDA to ban it in the U.S. as well.[6]

Sources: Sandwich breads, buns, rolls, and other baked goods.

BHA (Butylated Hydroxyanisole)

What it is: Synthetic preservative.

Reasons to avoid: BHA is an endocrine disruptor, linked to cancer and tumors in animal studies.[7] The International Agency for Research on Cancer classifies BHA as "possibly carcinogenic to humans"; it's been deemed a "reasonably anticipated human carcinogen" by the USDA's National Toxicology Program.[8] It's also on EWG's Dirty Dozen list of food additives to avoid and is banned in other countries.[9]

Sources: Sausage, pepperoni, pizza, canned soup, boxed potatoes, potato chips, drink mixes, canned refried beans, spaghetti sauce, and chewing gum.

BHT (BUTYLATED HYDROXYTOLUENE)

What it is: Synthetic preservative.

Reasons to avoid: BHT has been shown to affect the signaling from our gut to our brain that normally tells us to stop eating.[10] Disruptions in these signals could contribute to overeating and obesity. BHT is also an endocrine disruptor that is linked to cancer in some animal studies. The EWG includes BHT on its Dirty Dozen list of food additives to avoid.

Sources: Cereal, packaged nuts, pepperoni, cake mix, and granola bars.

BLUE #1 (BRILLIANT BLUE)

What it is: Artificial blue dye derived from petroleum.

Reasons to avoid: This is one of the worst artificial colors because it has been shown to cross the blood-brain barrier. According to testimony at an FDA committee meeting, the FDA asked doctors to stop adding Blue #1 to tube feedings because "patients were dying, not from their disease, but from the Blue number 1, which apparently caused refractory hypotension and metabolic acidosis, and also, incidentally, turned their colons bright blue."[11] This dye is also linked to hyperactivity and an increased risk of kidney tumors. Some research suggests it is a potential neurotoxin.[12]

Sources: Candy, drink mixes, soft drinks, chewing gum, toaster pastries, popsicles, marshmallows, fruit snacks.

CALCIUM PEROXIDE

What it is: Bleach and dough conditioner.

Reasons to avoid: If you see this chemical on an ingredients list, it's a sure sign that the food is heavily processed. It has been banned in Europe, as well as from some stores such as Whole Foods in the U.S.

Sources: Croutons, sandwich breads, buns, rolls, and other baked goods.

CALCIUM PROPIONATE

What it is: Mold inhibitor.

Reasons to avoid: Although this chemical is considered a safer preservative, research published in the *Journal of Paediatrics and Child Health* links it to "irritability, restlessness, inattention and sleep disturbance in some children."[13] Long-term consumption has been shown to damage the stomach lining and induce ulcers.

Sources: Croutons, sandwich breads, buns, rolls, and other baked goods.

CANOLA OIL

What it is: Refined cooking oil.

Reasons to avoid: Whenever I see the chefs on Food Network using canola oil I want to scream at the TV. . . and I have to admit, I sometimes do. For years, I was misled into thinking that canola oil was healthy and I would buy quarts of it. It's not healthy. This oil goes through intense processing with chemical solvents, steamers, neutralizers, de-waxers, bleach, and deodorizers before it ends up in the bottle. It is most often extracted with the neurotoxin hexane, and some hexane residue can remain in the oil. The FDA doesn't require food manufacturers to test for residues.

Canola oil is extracted from rapeseed plants that have been bred to have lower levels of toxic erucic acid, which causes heart damage in lab animals.[14] Before it was bred this way, it was called rapeseed oil and used for industrial purposes. It later got the fancy new name "canola," but it still contains trace amounts of erucic acid (up to 2 percent, which is considered "safe"). In 1995, conventional farmers began genetically engineering (GMO) rapeseed to be resistant to herbicides, and now almost all canola crops in North America are GMO. Research has also found some trans fat in canola oil, created during its heavy processing;[15] these trans fats are not labeled.

Sources: Boxed mixes, bakery items, desserts, dressings, sauces, frozen meals, crackers, and snack foods.

CARAMEL COLOR

What it is: Brown food coloring.

Reasons to avoid: Linked to cancer,[16] caramel color has no nutritional benefits and is only used cosmetically to improve the appearance of food. It's sometimes added unnecessarily to food and drinks that are naturally brown.

Sources: Soft drinks, pancake syrup, coffee shop drinks, cereal, deli meat, and soups.

CARRAGEENAN

What it is: Thickener and emulsifier to keep ingredients from separating.

Reasons to avoid: Known to cause digestive problems and intestinal inflammation, this additive can be contaminated with "degraded carrageenan." Tests have found as much as 25 percent degraded carrageenan in "food-grade carrageenan" (the kind used in food and drinks). Degraded carrageenan is classified as a "possible human carcinogen" by the International Agency for Research on Cancer.[17]

Sources: Almond milk, coconut milk, soy milk, dairy-free milks, ice cream, deli meat, cottage cheese, and coffee creamers.

CELLULOSE

What it is: Anti-caking agent and thickener usually made from wood. It is also sometimes used to bulk up foods with fake fiber.

Reasons to avoid: Cellulose is much cheaper to obtain from wood than from vegetables, so the food industry usually relies on wood by-products to make it. Cellulose can also come from vegetables, but will be listed on the label as such (very rare). Research links consumption of this additive (not naturally occurring) to weight gain, inflammation, and digestive problems.

Sources: Shredded cheese, pizza, spice mixes, pancake syrup, and foods labeled as "high fiber" or "added fiber."

CITRIC ACID

What it is: Preservative and flavor (sour taste).

Reasons to avoid: Although citric acid is naturally found in lemons and other fruits, the additive used in packaged foods is typically derived from mold made with GMO corn (not from fruit).[18]

Sources: Juice, bottled iced tea, citrus-flavored sodas, energy drinks, baby food, flavored chips, candy, and canned tomatoes.

CORN OIL

What it is: Refined cooking oil.

Reasons to avoid: Here's another oil that is processed with chemical solvents, steamers, neutralizers, de-waxers, bleach, deodorizers, and hexane. Unless it is Non-GMO Project verified or organic, corn oil typically comes from GMO corn.

Sources: Chips, frozen meals, coated pretzels, cookies, sausages, snack mix, crackers, microwave popcorn, canned soups, and canned chili.

CORN SYRUP

What it is: Heavily processed form of sugar made from corn.

Reasons to avoid: This refined sugar has no nutritional value. Unless the product is organic or Non-GMO Project verified, it is typically made from GMO corn that produces its own insecticide.

Sources: Sauces, crackers, desserts, pie, and pancake syrup.

Cottonseed Oil

What it is: Refined cooking oil.

Reasons to avoid: This oil is made from a by-product of industrial waste from the cotton farming industry (cotton isn't even a food crop). Despite being one of the most prevalent GMO crops, cotton crops are exposed to many agricultural chemicals and pesticides—which is why cotton has been called the "World's Dirtiest Crop."[19] Residues from these pesticides can potentially remain in cottonseed oil, according to data collected by the FAO/WHO Joint Meetings on Pesticides Residues.[20] To extract the oil, the cottonseeds are subjected to intensive chemical refining with toxic hexane, bleach, and deodorizers.

Sources: Fries, fried foods, chips, and baked goods.

DATEM (Diacetyl Tartaric Acid Esters of Monoglycerides)

What they are: Dough conditioner that is usually derived from soybean or canola oil (GMO crops).

Reasons to avoid: This ingredient can be a hidden form of deadly trans fat. See "Monoglycerides" below.

Sources: Sandwich breads, buns, baked goods, and crackers.

Dextrose

What it is: Heavily processed form of sugar, usually made from corn. It is also used as a filler.

Reasons to avoid: This refined sugar has no nutritional value. Unless the product is organic or Non-GMO Project verified, it is typically made from GMO corn that produces its own insecticide.

Sources: Chips, artificial sweeteners, frozen meals, cake mix, cookies, cereal, and meat sticks.

DIMETHYLPOLYSILOXANE ("SILLY PUTTY" INGREDIENT)

What it is: Defoaming agent.

Reasons to avoid: There have been no major studies conducted on the safety of dimethylpolysiloxane in food by the FDA or the food industry since it was approved in 1998. The FDA allows it to be preserved with formaldehyde, a very toxic substance.[21]

Sources: French fries, deep-fried foods, yogurt, fountain drinks, and phase oil (a butter substitute used by some restaurants).

ENRICHED FLOUR AND BLEACHED FLOUR

What they are: Heavily processed flours with synthetic vitamins and minerals added.

Reasons to avoid: Flour can be treated with any of the 60 different chemicals approved by the FDA before it ends up on store shelves, including chemical bleach. The processing destroys nutrients, such as vitamin E and fiber. It has no nutritional value and is essentially dead food, so food makers "enrich" it with synthetic vitamins (niacin, reduced iron, thiamine mononitrate, riboflavin, folic acid) that are not from nature. (See "Synthetic Vitamins" below). Wheat has been heavily hybridized to make it easier for the food industry and is believed to be contributing to an increase in celiac disease,[22] and is often sprayed directly with Monsanto's Roundup herbicide.

Sources: Breads, buns, rolls, and other baked goods.

ERYTHRITOL

What it is: Sugar alcohol and low-calorie sweetener.

Reasons to avoid: It can wreak havoc on healthy gut bacteria, leading to a whole host of diseases. Erythritol can bring on diarrhea, stomach upset, and headache when consumed in "normal amounts."[23] It is also a powerful insecticide.

Like other artificial sweeteners, it can also increase your cravings, so you'll end up eating more food. Although this is a naturally occurring sugar that is sometimes found in fruit, food manufacturers don't actually use the natural stuff. Instead they usually start with GMO corn (unless organic or non-GMO verified) and then put it through a complex fermentation process to come up with chemically pure erythritol.

Sources: Stevia products, diet drinks, yogurt, and pudding cups.

GELLAN GUM, LOCUST BEAN GUM, AND GUAR GUM

What they are: Thickeners.

Reasons to avoid: These ingredients are known to cause stomach issues such as bloating and gas in people who have sensitive digestive systems.[24]

Sources: Almond milk, coconut milk, soy milk, nondairy milks and creamers, ice cream, and cottage cheese.

HIGH-FRUCTOSE CORN SYRUP (HFCS)

What it is: Heavily processed sweetener made from cornstarch. It contains more fructose than regular corn syrup.

Reasons to avoid: This sweetener increases appetite, promotes weight gain, and can lead to type 2 diabetes, heart disease, cancer, and dementia.[25] HFCS has been shown to especially contribute to type 2 diabetes in children.[26] One study also found it can be contaminated with toxic mercury.[27]

Sources: Soft drinks, pancake syrup, barbecue sauce, ketchup, cookies, breads, buns, frosting, and pies.

HFCS-90 (FRUCTOSE OR FRUCTOSE SYRUP)

What it is: Heavily processed sweetener made from cornstarch. It contains more fructose than high-fructose corn syrup. Regular HFCS contains up to 55 percent fructose, whereas

HFCS-90 has 90 percent fructose by weight. This is nine times more fructose than the average fruit.

Reasons to avoid: Excessive fructose in your diet is associated with obesity and cardiovascular disease. HFCS-90 is derived from corn starch, which is likely GMO. Some companies say that fructose is natural and comes from fruit, but this processed additive is typically derived from GMO corn. When HFCS-90 is used, the ingredient label won't indicate that "high-fructose corn syrup" is an ingredient; rather, it is deceptively labeled as "fructose" or "fructose syrup" without any reference to high-fructose corn syrup.

Sources: Yogurt, cereal, granola bars, and potato chips.

Maltodextrin

What it is: Heavily processed starch used as a filler, thickener, preservative, and sweetener.

Reasons to avoid: Maltodextrin negatively affects gut bacteria: a disruption that can put you at greater risk of disease.[28] It has no nutritional value—meaning it is not real food—and is used as a filler to artificially increase the volume of processed foods. Unless it is organic or Non-GMO Project verified, it is commonly from GMO corn. It is also a hidden form of MSG.

Sources: Potato chips, mac and cheese, frozen meals, powdered drink mixes, and pudding.

Monoglycerides and Diglycerides (Mono- and Diglycerides)

What they are: Emulsifiers that help keep ingredients from separating.

Reasons to avoid: These are made from oil by-products, including partially hydrogenated canola and soybean oils that contain artificial trans fat, making this additive a hidden source of trans fat in our food. They are permitted even in foods labeled as "0 grams of trans fat" because they are categorized as emulsifiers (not lipids) by the FDA. Artificial trans fat is correlated with an increased risk of type 2 diabetes and heart disease.

Sources: Ice cream sandwiches, low-fat ice cream, frozen yogurt, peanut butter, margarine, nondairy creamer, tortillas, and bread.

Monosodium Glutamate (MSG)

What it is: Artificial flavor enhancer.

Reasons to avoid: Purely used to increase food cravings and irresistibility, MSG is linked to headaches, obesity, depression, and mental disorders.[29] Besides the additive monosodium glutamate (MSG), the food industry sneaks in other additives—such as yeast extract and hydrolyzed proteins—that contain free glutamic acids, which are chief components of MSG.

Sources: Frozen meals, chips, dressings, soups, rice, and pasta mixes.

Natural Flavors

What they are: Flavors made from a proprietary mixture of chemicals derived from anything in nature.

Reasons to avoid: The only difference between natural and artificial flavors is that natural flavors come from substances found in nature. Natural flavors are used to make fake food taste real. Every flavor may contain up to 100 ingredients, including synthetic chemicals, propylene glycol as a solvent, and the preservative BHA,[30] as well as GMO-derived ingredients (unless organic or Non-GMO Project verified). Flavors can also include excitotoxins such as MSG.

Sources: Almost all processed foods.

Neotame

What it is: Artificial sweetener.

Reasons to avoid: Although neotame is relatively new and rarely used, some health experts warn that it is more harmful to our health than aspartame.[31] But its safety is still up in the air. It is often used in foods, along with other artificial sweeteners.

Sources: Diet juice, yogurt, chewing gum, diet soda, orange drink, and drink mixes.

PROPYLPARABEN (E216) OR METHYLPARABEN

What it is: Synthetic preservative.

Reasons to avoid: Parabens are endocrine-disrupting chemicals linked to breast cancer and reproductive problems.[32] EWG includes propylparaben on its Dirty Dozen list of top food additives to avoid.

Sources: Snack cakes, desserts, frosting, tortillas.

PARTIALLY HYDROGENATED OILS (ARTIFICIAL TRANS FAT)

What it is: Oil that has been solidified with chemical processing. These fats are typically made with GMO soybean, cottonseed, or canola oil.

Reasons to avoid: These oils are strongly correlated with an increased risk of type 2 diabetes and heart disease.[33] The Institute of Medicine says trans fats have "no known health benefit" and there is no safe level to eat. The FDA required all food manufacturers to remove partially hydrogenated oils by June 2018, but food companies can still petition the FDA for a special permit to continue using them.

Sources: Frosting, baked goods, nondairy creamers, cookies, and crackers.

PROPYL GALLATE

What it is: Synthetic preservative.

Reasons to avoid: Linked to increased risk of tumors and endocrine disruption, this chemical is on EWG's list of additives to avoid.[34]

Sources: Sausage, pizza, and stuffing mix.

RED #3 (ERYTHROSINE)

What it is: Artificial red dye derived from petroleum.

Reasons to avoid: Recognized as an animal carcinogen, Red #3 was banned from cosmetics in 1990, yet the FDA still permits it in food.

Commonly found in: Strawberry milk, baked goods, maraschino cherries, candy, and sausage casings.

RED #40 (ALLURA RED)

What it is: Artificial red dye derived from petroleum.

Reasons to avoid: The most popular artificial color used in the U.S., Red #40 is linked to hyperactivity in children.[35] Europe requires any food containing this dye to carry the warning label "May Have an Adverse Effect on Activity and Attention in Children." This is why many food companies use natural colors in Europe instead. Controversial research suggests this dye can accelerate the appearance of tumors.[36] It has no nutritional benefits and is only used cosmetically to improve the appearance of food.

Sources: Soft drinks, candy, cake, frosting, cookies, fruit cups, cherry filling, popsicles, toaster pastries, cereal bars, cereals, ice cream, yogurt, and drink mixes.

SODIUM BENZOATE (E211) OR POTASSIUM BENZOATE (E212)

What they are: Synthetic preservatives.

Reasons to avoid: When combined with either ascorbic acid (vitamin C) or erythorbic acid, these preservatives produce benzene, a known carcinogen.

Sources: Soft drinks, pickles, syrups, sauces, and salad dressing.

Sodium Nitrate and Sodium Nitrite

What they are: Synthetic preservatives.

Reasons to avoid: Both are linked to increased risk of cancer.

Sources: Deli meat, ham, sausage, hot dogs, bacon, jerky, and meat snacks.

Sodium Phosphate

What it is: Preservative.

Reasons to avoid: Sodium phosphate exists in practically all processed foods. If you take in phosphate additives often, they can lead to excessive levels of phosphate in the blood. This accumulation puts you at risk of chronic kidney disease, increased mortality, heart disease, and accelerated aging. The EWG warns that sodium phosphate is a top additive to avoid.

Sources: Cooked chicken, pudding, gelatin, mac and cheese, frozen desserts, frozen meals, soup, deli meat, and imitation cheese slices.

Soybean Oil

What it is: Refined cooking oil.

Reasons to avoid: Here we have one of the most unhealthy oils around. It increases the risk of obesity, inflammation, cardiovascular disease, cancer, and autoimmune diseases. Unless it's organic or Non-GMO Project verified, it's almost always made from GMO soybeans. When researchers tested GMO soybeans, they found that they contain high levels of residues from the herbicide glyphosate (Monsanto's Roundup), compared to non-GMO soybeans.[37] To extract the oil, the soybeans are subjected to intensive chemical refining with toxic hexane, bleach, and deodorizers.

Sources: Vegetable oil, salad dressing, crackers, cookies, baked goods, trail mix, potato chips, frozen meals, frozen desserts, buns, soup, and sauces.

Soy Protein Isolate

What it is: Heavily processed protein supplement made from soy flour that has fiber, fat, and nutrients removed.

Reasons to avoid: Soy can cause hormonal disruptions because it has estrogen-mimicking properties. It also has an abundance of phytic acid, which inhibits absorption of calcium and other vital minerals in the diet.[38] The soy protein is usually extracted with the neurotoxin hexane (and the final product may contain residues of hexane). Unless it's organic or Non-GMO Project verified, it's also almost always made from GMO soybeans.

Sources: Protein powder, protein shakes, protein bars, veggie burgers, veggie dogs, soup, and frozen meals.

Stevia Extract (Rebaudioside A or Reb A)

What it is: A low-calorie sweetener.

Reasons to avoid: This is not the same as whole stevia leaf that you can grow in your backyard. The extract is highly processed using a patentable chemical-laden process that includes about 40 steps to process the extract from the leaf, relying on chemicals like acetone, methanol, ethanol, acetonitrile, and isopropanol.[39] Some of these chemicals are known carcinogens. Most stevia formulations on the market also contain natural flavors, along with either erythritol or dextrose. Look for "whole leaf stevia" or an extract that contains no additional additives instead.

Sources: Soft drinks, coconut water, kombucha, bottled tea, protein drinks, protein bars, juice, and yogurt.

Sucralose (Splenda)

What it is: Artificial sweetener made by chlorinating sugar.

Reasons to avoid: Independent animal research links sucralose to leukemia.[40] It's also been shown that artificial sweeteners are doing little to help people lose weight and are actually linked to weight gain.

Sources: Chewing gum, diet sodas and drinks, iced tea, yogurt, pudding, and fruit cups.

SYNTHETIC VITAMINS

What they are: Lab-created vitamins made from a variety of sources like coal tar, petroleum, or GMOs. Examples include: vitamin A palmitate, thiamine (vitamin B1), riboflavin (vitamin B2), ascorbic acid (vitamin C), and folic acid.

Reasons to avoid: These vitamins differ from their natural counterparts, and thus aren't believed to be absorbed by your body as well as naturally present vitamins from whole food. They are often found in foods labeled "enriched" or "fortified." Some fortified foods have been found to have dangerously high levels of synthetic vitamins and minerals—especially for kids.

Sources: Cereal, bread, snack bars, protein drinks, meal replacements, supplements, milk.

TAPIOCA STARCH

What it is: Starch often used to replace wheat in gluten-free foods.

Reasons to avoid: Tapioca starch can be hard to avoid completely on a gluten-free diet—but it's something to be aware of and to limit in your diet. It is very high in carbohydrates but hardly contains any fiber, fat, protein, vitamins, or minerals, and basically just supplies empty calories that can spike blood sugar higher than refined sugar does.

Sources: Gluten-free bread, gluten-free tortillas, gluten-free baked goods, gluten-free crackers.

TBHQ (TERT-BUTYLHYDROQUINONE)

What it is: Synthetic preservative.

Reasons to avoid: TBHQ has been linked to vision disturbances, liver enlargement, childhood behavioral problems, stomach cancer, and most recently, to the rise in food allergies.

Research shows that TBHQ negatively affects "T-cells," which are important immune system defenders, in a way that promotes allergies to tree nuts, milk, eggs, wheat, and shellfish.[41] Banned for use in food in other countries, including Japan, TBHQ is on the Center for Science in the Public Interest's list as one of the worst food additives ever. This ingredient is not always on the label.

Sources: Crackers, cookies, microwave popcorn, peanut butter chocolates, pastries, biscuits, and frozen pizza.

TITANIUM DIOXIDE

What it is: Food color used to brighten and whiten.

Reasons to avoid: Microscopic particles (nanoparticles) of titanium dioxide are sometimes used to make white foods even whiter and brighter; however, it is not always labeled. According to Friends of the Earth, "In laboratory studies, nanoparticles of titanium dioxide have been found to be immunologically active, meaning they cause a reaction from the body's defensive system. Recent studies have indicated these particles may play an important role in the initiation or exacerbation of gastro-intestinal inflammation, by adsorbing bacterial fragments and then carrying them across the gastro-intestinal tract."[42]

Sources: Yogurt, cottage cheese, powdered sugar, candy, chewing gum, pudding, drink mixes, marshmallows, and mayonnaise.

VANILLIN

What it is: Artificial flavor (imitation vanilla) typically made from petrochemicals and wood pulp.

Why to avoid: A fake food and an artificial flavor, vanillin tricks your brain into believing that you are eating real vanilla. It also doesn't contain all of the health-building antioxidants found in real vanilla extract.

Sources: Milkshakes, ice cream, yogurt, protein shakes, and candy.

Yellow #5 (Tartrazine) and Yellow #6 (Sunset Yellow)

What they are: Artificial yellow dyes derived from petroleum.

Reasons to avoid: Both are linked to several health issues, including allergies and hyperactivity in children.[43] Europe requires any food containing dyes to carry the warning label "May Have an Adverse Effect on Activity and Attention in Children." These dyes have been found to be contaminated with carcinogens, such as benzidine.[44] They have no nutritional benefits and are only used cosmetically to improve the appearance of food.

Sources: Candy, fruit snacks, cereals, mac and cheese, chips, and pickles.

Endnotes

Introduction

1. James, Susan Donaldson. "Subway Takes Chemical Out of Sandwich Bread After Protest." ABC News, February 5, 2014, National edition, Health section. http://abcnews.go.com/Health /subway-takes-chemical-sandwich-bread-protest/story?id=22373414.

2. Miller, Michael. "Kraft Mac & Cheese just got duller. You can thank (or blame) 'The Food Babe.'" *Washington Post*, April 21, 2015, U.S. edition, Morning Mix section. https://www.washingtonpost.com/news/morning -mix/wp/2015/04/21/kraft-mac-cheese-just-got-duller-you-can-thank-or -blame-the-food-babe/?utm_term=.f8538d1007ce.

3. Taylor, Kate. "How This Food Blogger Convinced Chick-fil-A to Go Antibiotics Free." *Entrepreneur*, February 12, 2014, U.S. edition, Franchises section. https://www.entrepreneur.com/article/231480#.

4. Daneshkhu, Scheherazade. "'Food Babe' Wins Battle with King of Beers." *Financial Times*, June 13, 2014, National edition. https://www.ft.com/ content/6fef0a00-f318-11e3-a3f8-00144feabdc0.

5. Taylor, Kate. "Can a Food Blogger Force Starbucks to Change Its Pumpkin Spice Latte?" *Entrepreneur*, August 27, 2014, U.S. edition. https://www .entrepreneur.com/article/236896.

6. U.S. Department of Health and Human Services, National Institutes of Health. Health, National Toxicology Program. NTP Technical Report on the Toxicology and Carcinogenesis Studies of 4-Methylimidazole (Cas No. 822-36-6) in F344/N Rats and B6C3F$_1$ Mice (Feed Studies). https://ntp .niehs.nih.gov/ntp/htdocs/lt_rpts/tr535.pdf.

7. Moyer, Justin. "Starbucks's Pumpkin Spice Latte now has pumpkin after shaming by the 'Food Babe.'" *Washington Post*, August 18, 2015, U.S. edition, Morning Mix section. https://www.washingtonpost.com/news/ morning-mix/wp/2015/08/18/starbuckss-pumpkin-spice-latte-now -has-pumpkin-after-shaming-by-jenny-mccarthy-of-food/?utm_term= .ecfb056f1451.

8. Rubin, Courtney. "Taking On the Food Industry, One Blog Post at a Time." *New York Times*, March 13, 2015, National edition, Style section. https:// www.nytimes.com/2015/03/15/style/taking-on-the-food-industry-one -blog-post-at-a-time.html.

9. University of Massachusetts Amherst, Department of Food Science. "Fergus M. Clydesdale," August 30, 2018. https://www.umass.edu/foodsci/faculty/fergus-m-clydesdale.

10. Sensient Technologies Corporation. "Leadership—Board of Directors." https://web.archive.org/web/20141226220528/http://www.sensient.com/about-us/leadership.

11. Sethness Products Company. "Serving Worldwide Markets with High Quality Caramel Color." Worldwide Locations. http://www.sethness.com/sethness-worldwide/.

12. Sensient Technologies Corporation. Schedule 14A, Definitive Proxy Statement, filed March 3, 2015. Sensient Technologies Corporation website. http://investor.sensient.com/static-files/ab2de4eb-ad87-41da-825a-1279743ced3b.

13. University of Massachusetts Amherst, Department of Food Science, "Fergus M. Clydesdale."

14. Ibid.

15. UCSF Industry Documents Library. "US Right to Know Agrichemical Documents." https://www.industrydocumentslibrary.ucsf.edu/chemical/collections/usrtk-agrichemical-collection/.

16. Algonquin College. "The School of Hospitality and Tourism at Algonquin College Presents an Evening with Dr. Joe Schwarcz: 'Demystifying the Science of Food,' Thursday, April 3, 2014, 5 pm Room H102, H Building, AC." http://www.algonquincollege.com/hospitalityandtourism/files/2014/03/Dr.-Joe-Schwartz-Poster.pdf.

17. UCSF Industry Documents Library, "US Right to Know Agrichemical Documents."

18. Pepperidge Farm Incorporated. "Our Story." https://www.pepperidgefarm.com/our-story/.

19. James, "Subway Takes Chemical Out of Sandwich Bread After Protest," ABC News.

20. Smith, Jack. "General Mills Starts Pulling Preservatives After Assault From Food Babe Army." *Observer*, February 6, 2015. http://observer.com/2015/02/general-mills-starts-pulling-preservatives-after-assault-from-food-babe-army/.

21. Ilan, Brat. "Panera to Drop at Least 150 Artificial Ingredients from Menu." *Wall Street Journal*, May 4, 2015, Business section. https://www.wsj.com/articles/panera-to-drop-at-least-150-artificial-ingredients-from-menu-1430787781.

22. Fuss, Sarah. "Activist Blogger 'Foodbabe' Scores Big Win With Chipotle." *Take Part*, March 27, 2013. https://web.archive.org/web/20130330101731/http://www.takepart.com/article/2013/03/27/blogger-foodbabe-win-chipotle-ingredients.

23. Ibid.

24. *Time* staff. "The 30 Most Influential People on the Internet." *Time*, March 5, 2015. http://time.com/3732203/the-30-most-influential-people-on-the-internet/.

25. Myers, Dan. "The 13 Most Powerful Women in Food." *The Daily Meal*, February 19, 2016. https://www.thedailymeal.com/eat/13-most-powerful-women-food-slideshow.

26. Berman, Rick. "The Crusade of Food Bimbos." *Washington Times*, April 23, 2015. https://www.washingtontimes.com/news/2015/apr/23/rick-berman-exposure-of-food-babe-dr-oz/.

Chapter 1

1. Newman, Andrew Adam. "Reminders That a Cookie Goes Beyond the Fig," *New York Times*, April 30, 2012. https://www.nytimes.com/2012/05/01/business/media/the-newtons-cookie-goes-beyond-the-fig.html.

2. U.S. Department of Health and Human Services, Public Health Service Agency for Toxic Substances and Disease Registry. "Toxicological Profile for N-Hexane." July 1999. https://www.atsdr.cdc.gov/toxprofiles/tp113.pdf; Yamamura, Yasuhiro. "n-Hexane polyneuropathy." *Psychiatry and Clinical Neurosciences* 23.1 (1969): 45–57. https://onlinelibrary.wiley.com/doi/abs/10.1111/j.1440-1819.1969.tb01441.x.

3. Canola Council of Canada. "Steps in Oil and Meal Processing." August 30, 2018. https://www.canolacouncil.org/oil-and-meal/what-is-canola/how-canola-is-processed/steps-in-oil-and-meal-processing; Gunnars, Kris . "Canola Oil: Good or Bad?" *Healthline Media*, March 9, 2014. https://www.healthline.com/nutrition/canola-oil-good-or-bad#section3.

4. Center for Science in the Public Interest. "In Europe, Dyed Foods Get Warning Label." July 20, 2010. https://cspinet.org/new/201007201.html.

5. Moss, Michael. "The Extraordinary Science of Addictive Junk Food." *The New York Times Magazine*, February 20, 2013. https://www.nytimes.com/2013/02/24/magazine/the-extraordinary-science-of-junk-food.html.

6. Hamerschlag, Kari, Anna Lappé, and Stacy Malkan. "Spinning Food: How food industry front groups and covert communications are shaping the story of food." Friends of the Earth. https://1bps6437gg8c169i0y1drtgz-wpengine.netdna-ssl.com/wp-content/uploads/wpallimport/files/archive/FOE_SpinningFoodReport_8-15.pdf.

7. The Center for Food Integrity. "Cracking the Code on Food Issues: Insights from Moms, Millennials and Foodies." The Center for Food Integrity 2014 Consumer Trust Research. http://www.foodintegrity.org/wp-content/uploads/2015/08/CFI2014ResearchBook.pdf.

8. Hamerschlag, Lappé, and Malkan, "Spinning Food."

9. Center for Food Safety. "Best Public Relations That Money Can Buy. A Guide to Food Industry Front Groups." May 2013. https://www.centerforfoodsafety.org/files/front_groups_final_84531.pdf.

10. Butler, Kiera. "How the US Government Helps McDonald's Sell Junk Food." *Mother Jones*, June 23, 2014. https://www.motherjones.com/environment/2014/06/usda-dairy-checkoff-mcdonalds-taco-bell/.

11. American Council on Science and Health. "About ACSH." https://www.acsh.org/about-acsh-0.

12. U.S. Right to Know. "Public Interest Groups to USA Today: Ditch Corporate Front Group Science Columns." News release, February 23, 2017. https://usrtk.org/news-releases/public-interest-groups-to-usa-today-ditch-corporate-front-group-science-columns/.

13. Malkan, Stacy. "Why is Cornell University hosting a GMO propaganda campaign?" *The Ecologist*, January 22, 2016. https://theecologist.org/2016/jan/22/why-cornell-university-hosting-gmo-propaganda-campaign.

14. Sustainable Pulse. "New York Farmers Ask Cornell University to Evict 'Alliance for Science' over GMO Bias." September 24, 2016. https://sustainablepulse.com/2016/09/24/new-york-farmers-ask-cornell-university-to-evict-alliance-for-science-over-gmo-bias/#.WwXf69MvyRv.

15. Cornell Alliance for Science. "Partners." https://web.archive.org/web/20170330031902/.

16. International Service for the Acquisition of Agri-biotech Applications (ISAAA). "Donor Support Groups." http://www.isaaa.org/inbrief/donors/default.asp.

17. Sustainable Pulse, "New York Farmers Ask Cornell University to Evict 'Alliance for Science' over GMO Bias," September 24, 2016.

18. Cornell Alliance for Science. "Cornell Alliance for Science Launches Global Ag Journalism Fellowship." News release, June 10, 2015.

19. The Center for Food Integrity. "CFI Members." http://www.foodintegrity.org/about/members/cfi-members/.

20. Malkan, Stacy. "Center for Food Integrity Partners with Monsanto." U.S. Right to Know, May 31, 2018. https://usrtk.org/gmo/center-for-food-integrity-partners-with-monsanto/.

21. U.S. Farmers & Ranchers Alliance. "Earning Consumer Trust in U.S. Food & Agriculture." *AffiliatesInsert_Apr18_v1.*

22. Hamerschlag, Lappé, and Malkan, "Spinning Food."

23. U.S. Right to Know. "U.S. Farmers and Ranchers Alliance—key facts," Hall of Shame. January 21, 2015. https://usrtk.org/hall-of-shame/us-farmers-and-ranchers-alliance/.

24. Chase, Spencer. "USFRA to Ramp Up Its Food Company Outreach on GMOs." *Agri-Pulse*, October 31, 2016. https://www.agri-pulse.com/articles/7931-usfra-to-ramp-up-its-food-company-outreach-on-gmos.

25. Quinn, Erin and Chris Young. "Who needs lobbyists? See what big business spends to win American minds." *The Center for Public Integrity*, January 17, 2015. https://www.publicintegrity.org/2015/01/15/16596/who-needs-lobbyists-see-what-big-business-spends-win-american-minds.

26. Folta, Kevin. *Let's Drink Weed Killer, Not!* (Blog). http://kfolta.blogspot .com/2015/03/lets-drink-weed-killer.html.

27. Malkan, Stacy. "The Misleading and Deceitful Ways of Dr. Kevin Folta." U.S. Right to Know, August 1, 2018. https://usrtk.org/our-investigations/ kevin-folta/.

29. Folta, Kevin. *Food Babe Visits My University* (blog). http://kfolta.blogspot .com/2014/10/food-babe-visits-my-university.html.

30. UCSF Industry Documents Library, "US Right to Know Agrichemical Documents."

31. Ibid.

32. Ibid.

33. Hamblin, James. "The Food Babe: Enemy of Chemicals." *The Atlantic*, February 11, 2015, Health section. https://www.theatlantic.com/health/ archive/2015/02/the-food-babe-enemy-of-chemicals/385301/.

34. Rubin, "Taking On the Food Industry, One Blog Post at a Time," *New York Times*.

35. UCSF Industry Documents Library, "US Right to Know Agrichemical Documents."

36. Lipton, Eric. "Food Industry Enlisted Academics in G.M.O. Lobbying War, Emails Show." *The New York Times*, September 5, 2015. https://www .nytimes.com/2015/09/06/us/food-industry-enlisted-academics-in-gmo -lobbying-war-emails-show.html.

37. These emails can be found at the USRTK Agrichemical Industry Archive at UCSF: https://www.industrydocumentslibrary.ucsf.edu/chemical/results/#q =(collection%3A%22USRTK%20Agrichemical%20Collection%22)&h=%7B %22hideDuplicates%22%3Atrue%2C%22hideFolders%22%3Atrue%7D&su bsite=chemical&cache=true&count=1433.

38. Schweers, Jeff. "UF prof donates Monsanto grant to food pantry." *Gainesville Sun*, August 28, 2015, Sports section. http://www.gainesville.com/article/ LK/20150828/SPORTS/604134071/GS/.

39. Lesser, Lenard I. et al. "Relationship between Funding Source and Conclusion among Nutrition-Related Scientific Articles." *PLOS Medicine* 4.1 (February 9, 2007): e5. http://journals.plos.org/plosmedicine/ article?id=10.1371/journal.pmed.0040005.

40. American Association of University Professors. "Big Food, Big Agra, and the Research University." November–December 2010. https://www.aaup.org/ article/big-food-big-agra-and-research-university#.WwX2UdMvyRs.

41. Simon, Michele. "Nutrition Scientists on the Take from Big Food, June 2015." Eat Drink Politics. http://www.eatdrinkpolitics.com/wp-content/ uploads/ASNReportFinal.pdf.

42. Ruskin, Gary. "Did 24 Coke-Funded Studies on Childhood Obesity Fail to Disclose Coke's Influence?" U.S. Right to Know, News release, December 11, 2017. https://usrtk.org/news-releases/did-24-coke-funded-studies-on -childhood-obesity-fail-to-disclose-cokes-influence/.

43. North Carolina Consumers Council. "Kids Eat Right Seal Removed from Kraft Singles Packages Following Opposition." April 1, 2015.

44. PepsiCo. "Frito-Lay Announces New Resources to Make Gluten Free Snacking a Cinch." Press release, August 13, 2012. http://www.pepsico .com/live/pressrelease/frito-lay-announces-new-resources-to-make-gluten -free-snacking-a-cinch08132012.

45. Hari, Vani. "Are You Being Tricked By These Food Industry Marketing Tactics?" *Food Babe* (blog). https://foodbabe.com/ are-you-being-tricked-by-these-food-industry-marketing-tactics/.

46. Butler, Kiera. "I Went to the Nutritionists' Annual Confab. It Was Catered by McDonald's." *Mother Jones*, May 12, 2014, Environment section. https://www.motherjones.com/environment/2014/05/ my-trip-mcdonalds-sponsored-nutritionist-convention/; Dietitians for Professional Integrity. "Really?! McDonald's Is Back as California Academy of Nutrition and Dietetics Sponsor." February 7, 2017. https://integritydietitians.org/2017/02/07/ really-mcdonalds-back-california-academy-nutrition-dietetics-sponsor-2/.

47. Moye, Jay. "Just the Facts: 10 Years In, Beverage Institute for Health & Wellness Expands Its Reach." December 17, 2014. https://www.coca -colacompany.com/stories/just-the-facts-10-years-in-beverage-institute-for -health-wellness-expands-its-reach.

48. Zelman, Kathleen. "17 Best Foods for Dieters." WebMD. https://www .webmd.com/diet/obesity/features/17-best-foods-for-dieters#1.

49. MyPlate. "All about the Dairy Group." U.S. Department of Agriculture, August 31, 2018. https://www.choosemyplate.gov/dairy.

50. Physicians Committee for Responsible Medicine. "Doctors Not Lovin' USDA-McDonald's Partnership to Push Disease-Causing Dairy." News release, April 3, 2018.

51. MacDonald, Lauren et al. "A Systematic Review and Meta-Analysis of the Effects of Pasteurization on Milk Vitamins, and Evidence for Raw Milk Consumption and Other Health-Related Outcomes." *Journal of Food Protection* 74, no. 11 (May 2011): 1814–32. https://www.ncbi.nlm.nih.gov/ pubmed/22054181.

52. Thielman, Sam and Dominic Rushe. "Government-Backed Egg Lobby Tried to Crack Food Startup, Emails Show." *The Guardian*, September 2, 2015, Business section. https://www.theguardian.com/us-news/2015/sep/02/ usda-american-egg-board-hampton-creek-just-mayo.

53. Gillam, Carey. "EPA Bows to Chemical Industry in Delay of Glyphosate Cancer Review." *Huffington Post,* October 19, 2016. https://www .huffingtonpost.com/carey-gillam/epa-bows-to-chemical -indu_b_12563438.html.

54. American Cancer Society. "Kenneth Portier, PhD, Managing Director, Statistics and Evaluation Center, American Cancer Society." *Expert*

Voices (Blog), August 31, 2018. http://blogs.cancer.org/expertvoices/ kenneth-portier.

55. CropLife America to Environmental Protection Agency. Letter. October 12, 2016. http://191hmt1pr08amfq62276etw2.wpengine.netdna -cdn.com/wp-content/uploads/2016/01/CLA-Comments-on-SAP -Disqualification-10-12-16.pdf.

56. Polansek, Tom. "U.S. EPA says glyphosate not likely to be carcinogenic to people." *Reuters*, December 20, 2017, Health News section. https://www .reuters.com/article/us-usa-pesticides-glyphosate/u-s-epa-says-glyphosate -not-likely-to-be-carcinogenic-to-people-idUSKBN1EE2XH.

57. Gillam, Carey. "FDA Suspends Testing for Glyphosate Residues in Food." *Huffington Post*, November 11, 2016. https://www.huffingtonpost.com/ carey-gillam/fda-suspends-glyphosate-r_b_12913458.html.

58. Staff and agencies. "Roundup weedkiller 'probably' causes cancer, says WHO study." *The Guardian*, March 21, 2015, Environment section. https://www.theguardian.com/environment/2015/mar/21/ roundup-cancer-who-glyphosate-.

Chapter 2

1. McNary, Chris. "Coke as a Healthy Treat? Company, Health Experts Get the Word Out." *Dallas Morning News*, March 16, 2015, Better Living section. https://www.dallasnews.com/life/healthy-living/2015/03/16/ coke-as-a-healthy-treat-company-health-experts-get-the-word-out.

2. Ibid.

3. Thacker, Paul. "Coca-Cola's secret influence on medical and science journalists." *BMJ* 357 (2017): j1638. https://doi.org/10.1136/bmj.j1638.

4. May, Ashley. "Coconut Oil Isn't Healthy. It's Never Been Healthy." *USA Today*, June 16, 2017. https://www .usatoday.com/story/news/nation-now/2017/06/16/ coconut-oil-isnt-healthy-its-never-been-healthy/402719001/.

5. D'Souza, Karen. "Nutrition Experts Warn Coconut Oil Is on Par with Beef Fat, Butter." *Chicago Tribune*, June 19, 2017, Health section. http://www .chicagotribune.com/lifestyles/health/ct-coconut-oil-bad-fat-20170619 -story.html.

6. Hampson, Laura. "This Popular Health Food Is Worse for You than Pork Lard." *Daily Star*, June 19, 2017, Health section. https://www.dailystar.co.uk/health/623489/ Is-coconut-oil-for-you-making-you-fat-health-benefits.

7. Valente, Danielle. "Coconut Oil Isn't Healthy Because It Raises Cholesterol Levels." *Elite Daily*, June 19, 2017. https://www.elitedaily.com/social-news/ coconut-oil-actually-bad-for-you/1995512.

8. American Heart Association News. "Advisory: Replacing Saturated Fat with Healthier Fat Could Lower Cardiovascular Risks." American Heart Association, June 15, 2017.

9. Lauretti, Elisabetta and Domenico Praticò. "Effect of canola oil consumption on memory, synapse and neuropathology in the triple transgenic mouse model of Alzheimer's disease." *Scientific reports* 7.1 (2017): 17134. https://www.nature.com/articles/s41598-017-17373-3.

10. Hamley, Steven. "The Effect of Replacing Saturated Fat with Mostly N-6 Polyunsaturated Fat on Coronary Heart Disease: a Meta-Analysis of Randomised Controlled Trials." *Nutrition Journal* 16, no. 1 (May 19, 2017): 1. https://nutritionj.biomedcentral.com/articles/10.1186/s12937-017-0254-5.

11. Taubes, Gary. "Vegetable Oils, (Francis) Bacon, Bing Crosby, and the American Heart Association." June 17, 2017. http://garytaubes.com/vegetable-oils-francis-bacon-bing-crosby-and-the-american-heart-association/; Teicholz, Nina. "Don't believe the American Heart Assn.—butter, steak and coconut oil aren't likely to kill you." *Los Angeles Times*, July 23, 2017. http://www.latimes.com/opinion/op-ed/la-oe-teicholz-saturated-fat-wont-kill-you-20170723-story.html.

12. Ibid.

13. Ibid.

14. Ibid.

15. American Heart Association. "Certified Products Listed by Food Category," Heart-Check Food Certification Program. June 4, 2018. http://www.heart.org/idc/groups/heart-public/@wcm/@fc/documents/downloadable/ucm_474830.pdf.

16. Ibid.

17. Corliss, Julie. "Eating too much added sugar increases the risk of dying with heart disease." *Harvard Health Blog*. https://www.health.harvard.edu/blog/eating-too-much-added-sugar-increases-the-risk-of-dying-with-heart-disease-201402067021.

18. Ibid.

19. Harvard School of Public Health. "Eating processed meats, but not unprocessed red meats, may raise risk of heart disease and diabetes." Press release, May 17, 2010. https://www.hsph.harvard.edu/news/press-releases/processed-meats-unprocessed-heart-disease-diabetes/.

20. Horovitz, Bruce. "One thing NOT in Starbucks' pumpkin latte: pumpkin." *USA Today*, August 25, 2014, Money section. https://www.usatoday.com/story/money/business/2014/08/25/starbucks-pumpkin-spice-latte-food-babe-nutritionist/14578839/.

21. Fox News. "What's really in Starbucks' pumpkin spice latte?" *Fox & Friends*, September 2, 2014. http://video.foxnews.com/v/3762855144001/?#sp=show-clips.

22. Godoy, Maria. "Is the Food Babe a Fearmonger? Scientists Are Speaking Out." NPR, December 4, 2014, *The Salt* (Blog) section. https://www.npr.org/sections/thesalt/2014/12/04/364745790/food-babe-or-fear-babe-as-activist-s-profile-grows-so-do-her-critics.

23. Haro von Mogel, Karl. *Have you signed the #Science14 letter yet?* (Blog). https://www.biofortified.org/2015/03/have-you-signed-the-science14-letter-yet/.

24. Senapathy, Kavin. "3 Tactics Donald Trump Shares with Dr. Oz, The Food Babe, and Other Snake Oil Salesmen." *Forbes*, October 5, 2016 https://www.forbes.com/sites/kavinsenapathy/2016/10/05/3-tactics-donald-trump-shares-with-dr-oz-the-food-babe-and-other-snake-oil-salesmen/#46bc86630ae8.

25. Senapathy, Kavin. "The Food Babe Is a Bully and Cotton Incorporated Isn't Going To Take It." *Forbes*, May 27, 2016. https://www.forbes.com/sites/kavinsenapathy/2016/05/27/the-food-babe-is-a-bully-cotton-incorporated-isnt-going-to-take-it/#353ccfac2fc0.

26. Senapathy, Kavin. "Del Monte Joins Food Babe Army, Shuns Fruit-Saving Technology." *Forbes*, April 5, 2016. https://www.forbes.com/sites/kavinsenapathy/2016/04/05/del-monte-joins-food-babe-army-shuns-fruit-saving-technology/#6bddd3f8638a.

27. Senapathy, Kavin. "The Toxic 'Chemical Hypocrisy' of Food Babe, Joseph Mercola and Mark Hyman," *Forbes*, December 3, 2015. https://www.forbes.com/sites/kavinsenapathy/2015/12/03/the-toxic-chemical-hypocrisy-of-food-babe-joseph-mercola-and-mark-hyman/#7bdea2ca2df6.

28. U.S. Right to Know, "U.S. Farmers and Ranchers Alliance—key facts," January 21, 2015.

29. "Monsanto transfers some cotton technology to Cotton Inc." *St. Louis Business Journal*, August 9, 2002. https://www.bizjournals.com/stlouis/stories/2002/08/05/daily76.html.

30. Kim, Danny. "Monsanto Emails Raise Issue of Influencing Research on Roundup Weed Killer." *New York Times*, August 1, 2017, Business section. https://www.nytimes.com/2017/08/01/business/monsantos-sway-over-research-is-seen-in-disclosed-emails.html.

31. Ibid.

32. Talking Biotech. "Sponsors." http://talkingbiotech.com/sponsors/.

33. CropLife Canada. "Members." August 31, 2018. https://croplife.ca/about-us/members-2/.

34. American Seed Trade Association. "About ASTA—Leadership." August 31, 2018. https://www.betterseed.org/about-asta/leadership/.

35. Food &Water Watch. "The Farm Bureau's Billions: The Voice of Farmers or Agribusiness?" July 2010. https://www.panna.org/sites/default/files/FWW_FarmBureau.pdf.

36. Manitoba Canola Growers Association. "Canola Check Off." August 31, 2018. https://canolagrowers.com/about-mcga/canola-check-off/.

37. Folta, Kevin. "160731 Folta total." https://drive.google.com/file/d/0B0GH8K8D3PEuTUJCa3Y5WkNxZEk/view.

38. Farm & Food Care Saskatchewan. "Members & Sponsors." https://farmfoodcaresk.org/about-us/members-and-sponsors/.

39. Great Lakes Crop Summit. "Sponsors." http://www.greatlakescropsummit
.com/sponsors.

40. Malkan, Stacy. "The Misleading and Deceitful Ways of Dr. Kevin Folta." U.S.
Right to Know, August 1, 2018. https://usrtk.org/our-investigations/kevin
-folta/. Bayer AG to Kevin Folta. Letter. May 21, 2017. https://usrtk.org/
wp-content/uploads/2017/10/Bayer_Folta_funding.pdf.

41. UCSF Industry Documents Library, "US Right to Know Agrichemical
Documents."

42. Knutson, Jonathan. "Agweek visits Monsanto: Touring the company's
biggest research center." *AgWeek*, Aug 8, 2016, Technology section. https://
www.agweek.com/business/technology/4089872-video-agweek-visits
-monsanto-touring-companys-biggest-research-center.

43. Rosenbloom, Cara. "A Diet Rich in Fruits and Vegetables Outweighs the
Risks of Pesticides." *Washington Post,* January 18, 2017, Lifestyle section.
https://www.washingtonpost.com/lifestyle/wellness/a-diet-rich-in-fruits
-and-vegetables-outweighs-the-risks-of-pesticides/2017/01/13/f68ed4f6
-d780-11e6-9a36-1d296534b31e_story.html?utm_term=.4971a66ea9c1.

44. Words to Eat By. "Services." http://wordstoeatby.ca/.

45. Rosenbloom, Cara. "A Diet Rich in Fruits and Vegetables Outweighs the
Risks of Pesticides." *Washington Post.*

46. Environmental Working Group. "Dirty Dozen: EWG's 2018 Shopper's Guide
to Pesticides in Produce." https://www.ewg.org/foodnews/dirty-dozen.php
.Environmental Working Group. "OUT NOW: EWG's 2018 Shopper's Guide
to Pesticides in Produce." https://www.ewg.org/foodnews/press.php.

47. Attkisson, Sharyl. "Astroturf and manipulation of media messages." Filmed
in January 2015 at University of Nevada. TEDx video, 10:36. https://www
.youtube.com/watch?v=-bYAQ-ZZtEU.

48. Experience Life staff. "Turf Wars." *Experience Life,* October 2015. https://
experiencelife.com/article/turf-wars/.

49. Ibid.

50. In Re: Roundup Products Liability Litigation,16-md-02741-VC (N.D.
Cal. 2016). https://www.cand.uscourts.gov/VC/roundupmdl. RT
staff, "Monsanto accused of hiring army of trolls to silence online
dissent—court papers." RT, May 2, 2017. https://www.rt.com/
usa/386858-monsanto-hired-trolls-court/.

51. Hari, Vani. "The Unethical Tactics Of The Chemical Industry
To Silence The Truth." *Food Babe* (blog). https://foodbabe.com/
the-unethical-tactics-of-the-chemical-industry-to-silence-the-truth/.

52. U.S. Right to Know. "GMO Answers Is a Crisis
Management PR Tool for GMOs & Pesticides." Food For
Thought, GMOs. March 1, 2018. https://usrtk.org/gmo/
gmo-answers-is-a-marketing-and-pr-website-for-gmo-companies/.

53. Szalavitz, Maia. "Mayo Clinic vs. WebMD: Another Perspective." *Time,*
February 7, 2011, Pharmaceuticals section. http://healthland.time
.com/2011/02/07/mayo-clinic-vs-webmd-another-perspective/.

54. WebMD. "A Bigger Discussion About Food." http://www.webmd.com/food -discussion/default.htm Internet archive.

55. Drake, Lisa to Kevin Folta. E-mail, January 2015. https://www.motherjones .com/wp-content/uploads/webmd.pdf.

56. Pinsker, Joe. "The Covert World of People Trying to Edit Wikipedia—for Pay: Can the Site's Dwindling Ranks of Volunteer Editors Protect Its Articles from the Influence of Money?" *The Atlantic,* August 11, 2015, Business section. https://www.theatlantic.com/business/archive/2015/08/ wikipedia-editors-for-pay/393926/.

57. Ibid.

Chapter 3

1. Associated Press. "Coke, Pepsi dropping controversial 'BVO' from all drinks." *USA Today*, May 5, 2014, News section. https://www.usatoday.com/story/news/nation/2014/05/05/ coke-pepsi-dropping-bvo-from-all-drinks/8736657/.

2. Quaker Instant Oatmeal Strawberries & Cream ingredients: Whole Grain Rolled Oats, Sugar, Creaming Agent (Maltodextrin, Sunflower And Palm Oils, Whey, Sodium Caseinate), Flavored And Colored Fruit Pieces (Dehydrated Apples [Treated With Sodium Sulfite To Promote Color Retention], Artificial Strawberry Flavor, Citric Acid, Red 40), Salt, Guar Gum, Artificial Flavor, Citric Acid, Niacinamide, Vitamin A Palmitate, Reduced Iron, Pyridoxine Hydrochloride, Riboflavin, Thiamin Mononitrate, Folic Acid.

3. Center for Science in the Public Interest, "In Europe, Dyed Foods Get Warning Label," July 20, 2010.

4. General Mills. "Red Velvet Cake Mix." Betty Crocker U.K. https://www .bettycrocker.co.uk/products/red-velvet-cake-mix.

5. Szabo, Liz. "Americans die younger than others in rich nations." *USA Today*, January 10, 2013, News section. https://www.usatoday.com/story/news/ nation/2013/01/09/americans-health-mortality-illness/1818903/; National Academies of Sciences, Engineering, and Medicine, Health and Medicine Division. "U.S. Health in International Perspective: Shorter Lives, Poorer Health." January 9, 2013. http://www.nationalacademies.org/hmd/ Reports/2013/US-Health-in-International-Perspective-Shorter-Lives-Poorer -Health.aspx.

6. Khazan, Olga. "A Shocking Decline in American Life Expectancy." *The Atlantic*, December 21, 2017, Health section. https://www.theatlantic.com/ health/archive/2017/12/life-expectancy/548981/.

7. The National Institute of Diabetes and Digestive and Kidney Diseases, Health Information Center. "Overweight & Obesity Statistics." August 2017. https://www.niddk.nih.gov/health-information/health-statistics/ overweight-obesity.

8. Centers for Disease Control and Prevention. "Childhood Obesity Facts." August 13, 2018. https://www.cdc.gov/obesity/data/childhood.html.

9. Berlinger, Joshua. "1 in 5 people will be obese by 2025, study says." *CNN*, April 1, 2016. https://www.cnn.com/2016/04/01/health/global-obesity -study/index.html.

10. Kindy, Kimberly. "Food Additives on the Rise as FDA Scrutiny Wanes." *Washington Post,* August 17, 2014, National Section. https://www .washingtonpost.com/national/food-additives-on-the-rise-as-fda-scrutiny -wanes/2014/08/17/828e9bf8-1cb2-11e4-ab7b-696c295ddfd1_story. html?utm_term=.469f1defb159.

11. Neltner, T., M. Maffini, and Natural Resources Defense Council. "Generally Recognized as Secret: Chemicals Added to Food in the United States." https://www.nrdc.org/sites/default/files/safety-loophole-for-chemicals-in -food-report.pdf.

12. Damewood, Kelly. "The GRAS Process: How Companies Legally Add Ingredients to Food." *Food Business News,* January 30, 2014, Food Policy & Law section. http://www.foodsafetynews.com/2014/01/the-gras-process-how -companies-legally-add-ingredients-to-food/#.WxWqcVMvyRt; Eng, Monica. "Who Determines Safety of New Food Ingredients? Critics Say Manufacturers Are Too Often Making the Call on Their Own Products." *Chicago Tribune,* August 25, 2012. http://articles.chicagotribune.com/2012-08-25/health/ ct-met-food-ingredients-20120825_1_food-supply-pew-health-group-u-s-food.

13. Neltner, Maffini, and Natural Resources Defense Council, "Generally Recognized as Secret."

14. Kindy, "Food Additives on the Rise as FDA Scrutiny Wanes," *Washington Post.*

15. Ibid.

16. U.S. Government Accountability Office. "Food Safety: FDA Should Strengthen Its Oversight of Food Ingredients Determined to Be Generally Recognized as Safe (GRAS)." GAO-10-246: March 5, 2010. https://www.gao .gov/products/GAO-10-246.

Chapter 4

1. O'Connor, Anahad. "'Fed Up' Asks, Are All Calories Equal?" *Well—New York Times* (blog), May 9, 2015. https://well.blogs.nytimes.com/2015/05/09/ fed-up-asks-are-all-calories-equal/.

2. Hyman, Mark. *The Key to Automatic Weight Loss!* (Blog). *Dr. Hyman.* http:// drhyman.com/blog/2014/05/19/key-automatic-weight-loss/.

3. Gardner, Christopher D. et al. "Effect of Low-Fat vs Low-Carbohydrate Diet on 12-Month Weight Loss in Overweight Adults and the Association with Genotype Pattern or Insulin Secretion." *JAMA* 319, no. 7 (February 20, 2018): 667–79. https://jamanetwork.com/journals/jama/article -abstract/2673150; Armitage, Hanae. "Low-fat or low-carb? It's a draw, study finds." *Stanford Medicine,* February 20, 2018. https://med.stanford. edu/news/all-news/2018/02/low-fat-or-low-carb-its-a-draw-study-finds. html.

4. Walters, D. Eric. "Aspartame, a sweet-tasting dipeptide." The Chicago Medical School Molecule of the Month, February 2001. http://www.chm.bris .ac.uk/motm/aspartame/aspartameh.html; Yoquinto, Luke. "The Truth About Aspartame." *Live Science*, April 13, 2012. https://www.livescience .com/36257-aspartame-health-effects-artificial-sweetener.html.

5. Fowler, S. P. et al. "Fueling the obesity epidemic? Artificially sweetened beverage use and long-term weight gain." *Obesity*, 16(8), August 2008, 1894–1900. https://www.ncbi.nlm.nih.gov/pubmed/18535548.

6. De Koning, Lawrence et al. "Sweetened Beverage Consumption, Incident Coronary Heart Disease and Biomarkers of Risk in Men." *Circulation* 125, no. 14, March 12, 2012: 1735–41. https://www.ncbi.nlm.nih.gov/ pubmed/22412070.

7. Swithers, Susan E. and Terry L. Davidson. "A role for sweet taste: calorie predictive relations in energy regulation by rats." *Behavioral Neuroscience* 122.1 (2008): 161. https://www.ncbi.nlm.nih.gov/ pubmed/18298259.

8. Swithers, Susan E., Chelsea R. Baker, and T. L. Davidson. "General and persistent effects of high-intensity sweeteners on body weight gain and caloric compensation in rats." *Behavioral Neuroscience* 123.4 (2009): 772. https://www.ncbi.nlm.nih.gov/pubmed/19634935.

9. Green, Erin and Claire Murphy. "Altered processing of sweet taste in the brain of diet soda drinkers." *Physiology & Behavior* 107.4 (2012): 560–67. https://www.ncbi.nlm.nih.gov/pmc/articles/PMC3465626/.

10. Elmhurst College. "Cellulose," Virtual Chembook. http://chemistry .elmhurst.edu/vchembook/547cellulose.html.

11. Chassaing, Benoit et al. "Dietary emulsifiers impact the mouse gut microbiota promoting colitis and metabolic syndrome." *Nature* 519.7541 (2015): 92–96. https://www.ncbi.nlm.nih.gov/pubmed/25731162.

12. Young, Chris. "Critic of Artificial Sweeteners Pilloried by Industry-Backed Scientists: Conflicts Abound among Industry's Defenders, Even on National TV." The Center for Public Integrity, August 6, 2014. https://www.publicintegrity.org/2014/08/06/15207/ critic-artificial-sweeteners-pilloried-industry-backed-scientists.

13. Ruskin, Gary. "Calorie Control Council (CCC)—key facts." U.S. Right to Know, January 17, 2015. https://usrtk.org/sweeteners/ calorie-control-council/.

14. Young, Chris. "Critic of Artificial Sweeteners Pilloried by Industry-Backed Scientists." The Center for Public Integrity, August 6, 2014.

15. U.S. Centers for Disease Control. "Prevalence of Overweight, Obesity, and Extreme Obesity Among Adults: United States, Trends 1960–1962 Through 2007–2008." https://www.cdc.gov/nchs/data/hestat/obesity_adult_07_08/ obesity_adult_07_08.pdf.

16. "U.S. News Reveals Best Diets Rankings for 2018." *U.S. News and World Report,* January 3, 2018. https://www.usnews.com/info/blogs/press-room/ articles/2018-01-03/us-news-reveals-best-diets-rankings-for-2018.

17. The Cornucopia Institute. "The Organic Watergate—White Paper. Connecting the Dots: Corporate Influence at the USDA's National Organic Program." https://www.cornucopia.org/USDA/OrganicWatergateWhitePaper.pdf.

18. Chassaing et al., "Dietary emulsifiers impact the mouse gut microbiota promoting colitis and metabolic syndrome," 92–96.

19. Center for Science in the Public Interest. "CSPI Downgrades Sucralose from 'Caution' to 'Avoid.' New Animal Study Indicates Cancer Risk." February 8, 2016. https://cspinet.org/new/201602081.html.

20. Holtcamp, Wendee. "Obesogens: An Environmental Link to Obesity." *Environmental Health Perspectives* 120, no. 2 (February 2012): a62–68. https://www.ncbi.nlm.nih.gov/pmc/articles/PMC3279464/.

21. National Institute of Environmental Health Sciences. "Endocrine Disruptors." May 2010. https://www.niehs.nih.gov/health/materials/endocrine_disruptors_508.pdf; Kristof, Nicholas. "Warnings from a Flabby Mouse." *New York Times*, January 19, 2013. https://www.nytimes.com/2013/01/20/opinion/sunday/kristof-warnings-from-a-flabby-mouse.html?mtrref=undefined&gwh=292B392FB3534BFC320B66C083F4C250&gwt=pay&assetType=opinion.

22. Chotiwat, C. et al. "Feeding a high-fructose diet induces leptin resistance in rats." *Appetite* 49, No. 1, (2007): 284. https://doi.org/10.1016/j.appet.2007.03.049; CBS/AP. "Fructose changes brain to cause overeating, scientists say." CBS News, January 2, 2013. https://www.cbsnews.com/news/fructose-changes-brain-to-cause-overeating-scientists-say/; Page, K. A. et al. "Effects of Fructose vs Glucose on Regional Cerebral Blood Flow in Brain Regions Involved With Appetite and Reward Pathways." *JAMA* 309, no.1 (2013): 63–70. https://doi:10.1001/jama.2012.116975.

23. Chamorro-García, R. et al. "Transgenerational Inheritance of Increased Fat Depot Size, Stem Cell Reprogramming, and Hepatic Steatosis Elicited by Prenatal Obesogen Tributyltin in Mice." *Environ Health Perspectives* 121, no. 3, (2013). https://www.ncbi.nlm.nih.gov/pubmed/23322813.

24. Phillips, Melissa Lee. "Phthalates and Metabolism: Exposure Correlates with Obesity and Diabetes in Men." *Environmental Health Perspectives* 115, no. 6 (2007): A312. https://www.ncbi.nlm.nih.gov/pmc/articles/PMC1892143/.

25. Melzer, David et al. "Association between Serum Perfluorooctanoic Acid (PFOA) and Thyroid Disease in the U.S. National Health and Nutrition Examination Survey." *Environmental Health Perspectives* 118, no. 5 (2010): 686–92. PMC. https://www.ncbi.nlm.nih.gov/pubmed/20089479.

26. Diep, Francie. "FDA Aims To Reduce Use Of Antibiotics For Fattening Farm Animals." *Popular Science*, December 11, 2013. https://www.popsci.com/article/science/fda-aims-reduce-use-antibiotics-fattening-farm-animals#_blank.

27. Katz, David L. and Stephanie Meller. "Can We Say What Diet Is Best for Health?" *Annual Review of Public Health* 35 (March 2014): 83–103. https://www.annualreviews.org/doi/full/10.1146/annurev-publhealth-032013-182351.

Chapter 5

1. McGandy, Robert B. et al. "Dietary fats, carbohydrates and atherosclerotic vascular disease." *New England Journal of Medicine* 277.4 (1967): 186–92. https://www.nejm.org/doi/full/10.1056/NEJM196707272770405.

2. Kearns, Cristin E., Dorie Apollonio, and Stanton A. Glantz. "Sugar industry sponsorship of germ-free rodent studies linking sucrose to hyperlipidemia and cancer: An historical analysis of internal documents." *PLOS Biology* 15.11 (2017): e2003460. https://journals.plos.org/plosbiology/article?id=10.1371/journal.pbio.2003460; O'Connor, Anahad. "How the Sugar Industry Shifted Blame to Fat." *New York Times*, September 12, 2016. https://www.nytimes.com/2016/09/13/well/eat/how-the-sugar-industry -shifted-blame-to-fat.html.

3. Yudkin, John. *Pure, White, and Deadly: How Sugar Is Killing Us and What We Can Do to Stop It.* New York: Penguin, 2013.

4. Ibid., 81–93.

5. Ibid., 110, 135–136.

6. Ibid., 81–93.

7. Ibid., 2.

8. Ibid., 167.

9. Taubes, Gary and Cristin Kearns Couzens. "Big Sugar's Sweet Little Lies." *Mother Jones*, November/December 2012. https://www.motherjones.com/environment/2012/10/sugar-industry-lies-campaign/.

10. U.S. Department of Agriculture. "A Brief History of USDA Food Guides." ChooseMyPlate.gov. https://www.choosemyplate.gov/brief-history-usda-food-guides.

11. Taubes, Gary. "Is Sugar Toxic?" *The New York Times Magazine*, April 13, 2011. https://www.nytimes.com/2011/04/17/magazine/mag-17Sugar-t.html.

12. Ibid.

13. New Hampshire Department of Health and Human Services. "How Much Sugar Do You Eat? You May Be Surprised!" https://www.dhhs.nh.gov/dphs/nhp/documents/sugar.pdf.

14. Taubes, "Is Sugar Toxic?," April 13, 2011.

15. Ibid.

16. Friedman, Richard. "What Cookies and Meth Have in Common." *New York Times*, June 30, 2017, Opinion section. https://www.nytimes .com/2017/06/30/opinion/sunday/what-cookies-and-meth-have-in -common.html.

17. Hyman, Mark. "7 Ways to Permanently Banish Belly Fat." *Dr. Hyman* (Blog). http://drhyman.comblog/2015/01/29/7-ways-permanently-banish-belly-fat/.

18. Ibid.

19. Hunter, Philip. "The Inflammation Theory of Disease: The Growing Realization That Chronic Inflammation Is Crucial in Many Diseases Opens

New Avenues for Treatment." *EMBO Reports* 13.11 (2012): 968–70. https://www.ncbi.nlm.nih.gov/pmc/articles/PMC3492709/.

20. Thuy, Sabine et al. "Nonalcoholic Fatty Liver Disease in Humans Is Associated with Increased Plasma Endotoxin and Plasminogen Activator Inhibitor 1 Concentrations and with Fructose Intake." *The Journal of Nutrition* 138, no. 8 (August 2008): 1452–55. https://academic.oup.com/jn/article/138/8/1452/4750797.

21. Maniam, Jayanthi et al. "Sugar Consumption Produces Effects Similar to Early Life Stress Exposure on Hippocampal Markers of Neurogenesis and Stress Response." *Frontiers in Molecular Neuroscience* 8, no. 86 (January 19, 2016). https://www.ncbi.nlm.nih.gov/pmc/articles/PMC4717325/.

22. Schmidt, Elaine. "This Is Your Brain on Sugar: UCLA Study Shows High-Fructose Diet Sabotages Learning, Memory. Eating More Omega-3 Fatty Acids Can Offset Damage, Researchers Say." UCLA Newsroom, May 15, 2012. http://newsroom.ucla.edu/releases/this-is-your-brain-on-sugar-ucla-233992.

23. Hanson, Nick. "Eating Lots of Carbs, Sugar May Raise Risk of Cognitive Impairment, Mayo Clinic Study Finds." Mayo Clinic news release, October 16, 2012. https://newsnetwork.mayoclinic.org/discussion/eating-lots-of-carbs-sugar-may-raise-risk-of-cognitive-impairment-mayo-clinic-study-finds/.

24. Sanchez, Albert et al. "Role of sugars in human neutrophilic phagocytosis." *The American Journal of Clinical Nutrition* 26, issue 11 (November 1, 1973): 1180–84. https://doi.org/10.1093/ajcn/26.11.1180.

25. DiNicolantonio, James J. et al. "Added Fructose: A Principal Driver of Type 2 Diabetes Mellitus and Its Consequences." *Mayo Clinic Proceedings* 90, no. 3 (March 2015): 372–81. https://www.ncbi.nlm.nih.gov/pubmed/25639270.

26. Hyman, Mark. "Eggs Don't Cause Heart Attacks—Sugar Does." *Dr. Hyman* (Blog). http://drhyman.com/blog/2014/02/07/eggs-dont-cause-heart-attacks-sugar/.

27. Ibid.

28. Tappy, Luc. "Q&A: 'Toxic' Effects of Sugar: Should We Be Afraid of Fructose?" *BMC Biology* 10, no. 42 (May 21, 2012). https://www.ncbi.nlm.nih.gov/pubmed/22613805.

29. Malkan, Stacy. "ILSI Wields Stealthy Influence for Food, Agrichemical Industries." U.S. Right to Know. June 28, 2016. https://usrtk.org/sweeteners/ilsi-wields-stealthy-influence-for-the-food-and-agrichemical-industries/.

30. Erickson, Jennifer et al. "The Scientific Basis of Guideline Recommendations on Sugar Intake: A Systematic Review." *Annals of Internal Medicine* 166, no. 4 (February 21, 2017): 257–67. http://annals.org/aim/fullarticle/2593601/scientific-basis-guideline-recommendations-sugar-intake-systematic-review; Choi, Candice. "Snickers maker criticizes industry-funded paper on sugar." *AP News*, December 21, 2016. https://apnews.com/cb26ddb939114d8ea0c219d27a788482.

31. Lustig, Robert H., Laura A. Schmidt, and Claire D. Brindis. "Public health: the toxic truth about sugar." *Nature* 482.7383 (2012): 27–29. https://www.ncbi.nlm.nih.gov/pubmed/22297952.

32. Friedman, Richard. "What Cookies and Meth Have in Common." *New York Times* June 30, 2017 Opinion section. https://www.nytimes.com/2017/06/30/opinion/sunday/what-cookies-and-meth-have-in-common.html.

33. Taubes and Couzens, "Big Sugar's Sweet Little Lies."

34. Taubes and Couzens, "Big Sugar's Sweet Little Lies."

35. Cohen, Deborah. "The Truth about Sports Drinks." *BMJ* 345 (July 18, 2012). https://www.bmj.com/content/345/bmj.e4737; Abrams, Lindsay. "The Controversial Science of Sports Drinks." *The Atlantic*, July 2012. https://www.theatlantic.com/health/archive/2012/07/the-controversial-science-of-sports-drinks/260124/.

36. Freeman, David. "Does Candy Keep Kids from Getting Fat?" CBS News, June 29, 2011, News section. https://www.cbsnews.com/news/does-candy-keep-kids-from-getting-fat/.

37. Choi, Candice. "Chocolate Milk Maker Wanted Study Touted with 'Concussion.'" *AP News*, April 20, 2016. https://apnews.com/24e44163938e4bf9a4c980ff76e7cab5/chocolate-milk-study-was-timed-concussion-movie.

38. Letzter, Rafi. "A Viral Story That Claimed Eating Ice Cream for Breakfast Will Make You Smarter Points to a Bigger Problem in Health Journalism." *Business Insider*, November 30, 2016. http://www.businessinsider.com/dont-eat-ice-cream-breakfast-2016-11.

39. Choi, Candice. "Can Breakfast Help Keep Us Thin? Nutrition Science Is Tricky." *Seattle Times*, January 19, 2017, Business section. https://www.seattletimes.com/business/can-breakfast-help-keep-us-thin-nutrition-science-is-tricky/.

40. Environmental Working Group. "Children's Cereals: Cereals Contain Far More Sugar Than Experts Recommend." May 15, 2014. https://www.ewg.org/research/childrens-cereals-sugar-pound/cereals-contain-far-more-sugar-experts-recommend#.W4WwuJNKiRs.

41. Smith, Aaron. "Cash-Strapped Farmers Feed Candy to Cows." CNN, October 10, 2012, Money section. http://money.cnn.com/2012/10/10/news/economy/farmers-cows-candy-feed/index.html.

42. U.S. Department of Agriculture. "2015–2020 Dietary Guidelines for Americans." https://www.cnpp.usda.gov/2015-2020-dietary-guidelines-americans.

43. Corn Refiners Association. "Sweeteners." http://www.corn.org/products/sweeteners/.

Chapter 6

1. Personal e-mail correspondence.

2. U.S. Department of Health and Human Services, National Institutes of Health, National Toxicology Program. "NTP Technical Report on The Toxicology And Carcinogenesis Studies Of 4-Methylimidazole (Cas No. 822-36-6) in F344/N Rats And B6c3f1 Mice (Feed Studies)."

3. International Agency for Research on Cancer. "Agents Classified by the IARC Monographs, Volumes 1–121." List of Classifications. http://monographs .iarc.fr/ENG/Classification/.

4. Consumer Reports. "Consumer Reports Test Results for 4-MEI in Soft Drinks." https://www.consumerreports.org/content/dam/cro/news_ articles/health/PDFs/CRO_Carmel_CompleteTestResults_1_14.pdf.

5. Fox News, "What's really in Starbucks' pumpkin spice latte?," *Fox & Friends*.

6. Giammona, Craig. "Starbucks Pulls Artificial Coloring From Pumpkin Spice Latte." *Bloomberg*, August 17, 2015, Business Section. https://www.bloomberg.com/news/articles/2015-08-17/ starbucks-pulls-artificial-coloring-from-pumpkin-spice-latte.

7. U.S. Department of Health and Human Services Centers for Disease Control and Prevention. "Get the Facts: Sugar-Sweetened Beverages and Consumption." https://www.cdc.gov/nutrition/data-statistics/sugar -sweetened-beverages-intake.html.

8. Fung, Teresa T. et al. "Sweetened Beverage Consumption and Risk of Coronary Heart Disease in Women." *The American Journal of Clinical Nutrition* 89, no. 4 (2009): 1037–42. https://www.ncbi.nlm.nih.gov/pmc/ articles/PMC2667454/.

9. Yang, Quanhe et al. "Added sugar intake and cardiovascular diseases mortality among US adults." *JAMA Internal Medicine* 174, no. 4 (2014): 516–24. https://jamanetwork.com/journals/jamainternalmedicine/ fullarticle/1819573.

10. Center for Science in the Public Interest. "CSPI Downgrades Sucralose from 'Caution' to 'Avoid.' New Animal Study Indicates Cancer Risk." February 8, 2016. https://cspinet.org/new/201602081.html.

11. Kobylewski, Sarah and Michael Jacobson. "Food Dyes: A Rainbow of Risks." Center for Science in the Public Interest, June 2010. https://cspinet.org/ resource/food-dyes-rainbow-risks.

12. Dos Santos, Vânia Paula Salviano et al. "Benzene as a Chemical Hazard in Processed Foods." *International Journal of Food Science* 2015, Article ID 545640 (2015). https://doi.org/10.1155/2015/545640.

13. Beverage Institute. "Move." The Coca-Cola Company, May 17, 2013. https:// www.coca-colacompany.com/stories/move.

14. Orlov, Alex. "Leaked emails reveal largest group of dietitians wants to hide ties to Big Soda." Mic, February 23, 2017. https://mic.com/articles/169224/ leaked-emails-reveal-largest-group-of-dietitians-wants-to-hide-ties-to-big -soda#.TpcKMgCPt; Tribune News Services. "Soda group suspends payments to dietitians opposing new tax." Chicago Tribune, October 6, 2016, Business section. http://www.chicagotribune.com/business/ct-soda-group-dietitians -20161006-story.html.

15. Cronin, Jeff and Ariana Stone. "Soda Industry Spent $67 Million Opposing State, City Soda Taxes & Warning Labels." Center for Science in the Public Interest, September 21, 2016. https://cspinet.org/news/soda-industry-spent -67-million-opposing-state-city-soda-taxes-warning-labels-20160921.

16. Aaron, Daniel G. et al. "Sponsorship of National Health Organizations by Two Major Soda Companies," *American Journal of Preventive Medicine* 52, no. 1 (January 2017): 20–30. https://www.ajpmonline .org/article/S0749-3797(16)30331-2/abstract; Fox, Maggie. "Have Soda Company Donations Influenced Health Groups?" *NBC News*, October 10, 2016. https://www.nbcnews.com/health/health-news/ have-soda-company-donations-influenced-health-groups-n663866.

17. O'Connor, Anahad. "Coca-Cola Funds Scientists Who Shift Blame for Obesity Away From Bad Diets," *Well—New York Times* (Blog). https://well .blogs.nytimes.com/2015/08/09/coca-cola-funds-scientists-who-shift -blame-for-obesity-away-from-bad-diets/.

18. Choi, Candice. "APNewsBreak: Emails reveal Coke's role in anti-obesity group." *AP News*, November 24, 2015. https://www.apnews.com/ce372c3d8 9d442a79458e6d32e713865.

19. Barlow, Pepita et al. "Science Organisations and Coca-Cola's 'War' with the Public Health Community: Insights from an Internal Industry Document." *Journal of Epidemiology & Community Health* (March 2018). http://jech.bmj .com/content/early/2018/03/14/jech-2017-210375.

20. O'Connor, Anahad. "Coca-Cola Funds Scientists Who Shift Blame for Obesity Away from Bad Diets." August 9, 2015; O'Connor, Anahad. "Coke Discloses Millions in Grants for Health Research and Community Programs." *Well—New York Times* (Blog), September 22, 2015. http://well .blogs.nytimes.com/2015/09/22/coke-discloses-millions-in-grants-for -health-research-and-community-programs/.

21. Pfister, Kyle. "The New Faces of Coke." Medium, September 28, 2015. https:// medium.com/cokeleak/the-new-faces-of-coke-62314047160f.

22. Ibid.

23. Gillam, Carey. "Beverage Industry Finds Friend inside U.S. Health Agency." *Huffington Post*, December 6, 2017. https://www.huffingtonpost.com/ carey-gillam/beverage-industry-finds-f_b_10715584.html; Gillam, Carey. "CDC Official Exits Agency after Coca-Cola Connections Come to Light." *Huffington Post*, June 30, 2016. https://www.huffingtonpost.com/carey -gillam/cdc-official-exits-agency_b_10760490.html; Gillam, Carey. "More Coca-Cola Ties Seen inside U.S. Centers for Disease Control." *Huffington Post*, August 1, 2016. https://www.huffingtonpost.com/carey-gillam/more -coca-cola-ties-seen_b_11287198.html.

24. UCSF Industry Documents Library, "US Right to Know Agrichemical Documents."

25. Nestle, Marion. "I've Been Wikileaked!" *Food Politics* (Blog), October 13, 2016. https://www.foodpolitics.com/2016/10/ive-been-wikileaked/.

Chapter 7

1. O'Connor, Anahad. "The Claim: Artificial Sweeteners Can Raise Blood Sugar." *New York Times*, July 19, 2010, U.S. Edition, Health section. https://www.nytimes.com/2010/07/20/health/20real.html?ref=health.

2. Hammond, H. C. "Is Maltodextrin Causing Your Blood Sugar Spikes?" *Diabetics Weekly*, June 29, 2017. https://diabeticsweekly.com/maltodextrin-causing-blood-sugar-spikes/.

3. Tobias, Deirdre et al. "Effect of Low-Fat vs. Other Diet Interventions on Long-Term Weight Change in Adults: A Systematic Review and Meta-Analysis." *The Lancet Diabetes & Endocrinology* 3, no. 12 (December 1, 2015): 968–79. https://www.thelancet.com/journals/landia/article/PIIS2213-8587(15)00367-8/abstract.

4. Schwingshackl, Lukas et al. "Comparison of Effects of Long-Term Low-Fat vs High-Fat Diets on Blood Lipid Levels in Overweight or Obese Patients: A Systematic Review and Meta-Analysis." *Journal of the Academy of Nutrition and Dietetics* 113, no. 12 (December 2013): 1640–61. https://www.ncbi.nlm.nih.gov/pubmed/24139973.

5. Mozaffarian, Dariush. "Dietary and Policy Priorities for Cardiovascular Disease, Diabetes, and Obesity: A Comprehensive Review." *Circulation* 133, no. 2 (January 12, 2016): 187–225. https://www.ncbi.nlm.nih.gov/pubmed/26746178.

6. U.S. Food and Drug Administration. "Final Determination Regarding Partially Hydrogenated Oils (Removing Trans Fat)." May 15, 2018. https://www.fda.gov/Food/IngredientsPackagingLabeling/FoodAdditivesIngredients/ucm449162.htm.

7. U.S. Food and Drug Administration. "FDA Takes Step to Further Reduce Trans Fats in Processed Foods." News release, Nov. 7, 2013. https://web.archive.org/web/20131110003708/https://www.fda.gov/NewsEvents/Newsroom/PressAnnouncements/ucm373939.htm.

8. U.S. Department of Health and Human Services. Genetics Home Reference. "Celiac Disease." https://ghr.nlm.nih.gov/condition/celiac-disease#statistics.

9. Celiac Disease Foundation. "Screening." https://celiac.org/celiac-disease/understanding-celiac-disease-2/diagnosing-celiac-disease/screening/.

10. Celiac Disease Foundation. "Celiac Disease Symptoms." https://celiac.org/celiac-disease/understanding-celiac-disease-2/celiacdiseasesymptoms/.

11. NPD Group, Inc. "Percentage of U.S. Adults Trying to Cut Down or Avoid Gluten in Their Diets Reaches New High in 2013, Reports NPD." News release, March 6, 2013. https://www.npd.com/wps/portal/npd/us/news/press-releases/percentage-of-us-adults-trying-to-cut-down-or-avoid-gluten-in-their-diets-reaches-new-high-in-2013-reports-npd/.

12. International Agency for Research on Cancer, "Agents Classified by the IARC Monographs, Volumes 1–121."

13. Consumer Reports. "Results of Our Tests of Rice and Rice Products." Consumer Reports Arsenic in Food, November 2012. https://www .consumerreports.org/content/dam/cro/magazine-articles/2012/November/ Consumer%20Reports%20Arsenic%20in%20Food%20November%20 2012_1.pdf.

14. International Agency for Research on Cancer, "Agents Classified by the IARC Monographs, Volumes 1–121."

15. Neslen, Arthur. "Glyphosate shown to disrupt microbiome 'at safe levels', study claims." *The Guardian*, May 16, 2018. https://www.theguardian.com/environment/2018/may/16/ glyphosate-shown-to-disrupt-microbiome-at-safe-levels-study-claims.

16. Wu, Jason et al. "Are Gluten-Free Foods Healthier Than Non-Gluten-Free Foods? An Evaluation of Supermarket Products in Australia." *British Journal of Nutrition* 114, no. 3 (August 14, 2015): 448–54. https://www.ncbi.nlm .nih.gov/pubmed/26119206.

17. Niewinski, Maryn. "Advances in Celiac Disease and Gluten-Free Diet." *Journal of the American Dietetic Association* 108, no. 4 (April 2008): 661–72. https://www.ncbi.nlm.nih.gov/pubmed/18375224.

18. Taillie, Lindsey Smith et al. "No Fat, No Sugar, No Salt . . . No Problem? Prevalence of 'Low-Content' Nutrient Claims and Their Associations with the Nutritional Profile of Food and Beverage Purchases in the United States." *Journal of the Academy of Nutrition and Dietetics* 117, no. 9 (September 2017): 1366–74. https://jandonline.org/article/ S2212-2672(17)30072-2/abstract.

Chapter 8

1. Environmental Working Group. "Synthetic Ingredients in Natural Flavors and Natural Flavors in Artificial Flavors." http://www.ewg.org/foodscores/ content/natural-vs-artificial-flavors#.Wwni49MvyRt.

2. International Agency for Research on Cancer, "Agents Classified by the IARC Monographs, Volumes 1–121."

3. Quinn, Erin and Chris Young. "Meet the Secret Group That Decides Which Flavors Are 'Natural.'" *Time*, June 9, 2015, Politics section. http://time .com/3913232/natural-flavoring-government/.

4. Center for Science in the Public Interest et al. to Center for Food Safety and Applied Nutrition. Letter. June 10, 2015. https://cspinet.org/sites/default/ files/attachment/food-additive-petition-2015.pdf.

5. Schatzker, Mark. *The Dorito Effect: The Surprising New Truth About Food and Flavor.* New York: Simon and Schuster, 2015.

6. Ibid.

7. *60 Minutes*. "The Flavorists: Tweaking Tastes and Creating Cravings." CBS News, November 27, 2011.

8. Andrews, David. "Synthetic Ingredients in Natural Flavors and Natural Flavors in Artificial Flavors." *Environmental Working Group.* https://www.ewg.org/foodscores/content/natural-vs-artificial-flavors.

9. Personal conversation, August 23, 2017.

10. Schatzker, *The Dorito Effect.*

11. Curwin, Brian et al. "Flavoring Exposure in Food Manufacturing." *Journal of Exposure Science & Environmental Epidemiology* 25.3 (2015): 324–33. https://www.ncbi.nlm.nih.gov/pmc/articles/PMC4520397/.

Chapter 9

1. Markel, Howard. "The remarkable history in your cereal bowl." *CNN*, August 13, 2017, Health section. https://www.cnn.com/2017/08/13/health/kellogg-corn-flakes-wellness-history-markel/index.html; Severson, Kim. "A Short History of Cereal." *The New York Times*, February 22, 2016, Food section. https://www.nytimes.com/interactive/2016/02/22/dining/history-of-cereal.html.

2. *Akron Beacon Journal* staff. "Akron experiment makes medical history." *Akron Beacon Journal*, March 8, 2009, Lifestyle section. https://www.ohio.com/akron/lifestyle/akron-experiment-makes-medical-history.

3. Ibid.

4. Institute of Medicine (US) Committee on Use of Dietary Reference Intakes in Nutrition Labeling. *Dietary Reference Intakes: Guiding Principles for Nutrition Labeling and Fortification. 3, Overview of Food Fortification in the United States and Canada.* Washington, DC: National Academies Press, 2003. https://www.ncbi.nlm.nih.gov/books/NBK208880/.

5. Crider, Krista S., Lynn B. Bailey, and Robert J. Berry. "Folic Acid Food Fortification—Its History, Effect, Concerns, and Future Directions." *Nutrients* 3.3 (2011): 370–84. https://www.ncbi.nlm.nih.gov/pmc/articles/PMC3257747/.

6. Ostrow, Ruth. "Vitamins and supplements—here are the chemicals you should know about." *The Australian*, August 14, 2015. https://www.theaustralian.com.au/life/health-wellbeing/vitamins-and-supplements--here-are-the-chemicals-you-should-know-about/news-story/d3fbda04ebfa45ee54912c5d87216321.

7. Burton, G. W. et al. "Human plasma and tissue alpha-tocopherol concentrations in response to supplementation with deuterated natural and synthetic vitamin E." *The American Journal of Clinical Nutrition* 67, Issue 4 (1998): 669–84. https://www.ncbi.nlm.nih.gov/pubmed/9537614.

8. Liu, Rui Hai. "Health benefits of fruit and vegetables are from additive and synergistic combinations of phytochemicals." *The American Journal of Clinical Nutrition* 78, Issue 3 (2003): 517S–520S. https://academic.oup.com/ajcn/article/78/3/517S/4689990.

9. Freuman, Tamara Duker. "When Nutrition Labels Lie." *U.S. News & World Report*, August 21, 2012, Health section. https://health.usnews.com/ health-news/blogs/eat-run/2012/08/21/when-nutrition-labels-lie.

10. Ibid.

11. Naidenko, O. and R. Sharp. "How Much is Too Much? Excess Vitamins and Minerals in Food Can Harm Kids' Health." Environmental Working Group. https://static.ewg.org/reports/2014/children_ at_risk/pdf/too_much_of_a_good_thing. pdf?_ga=2.33421689.691200960.1530124660-514613677.1510617920.

12. Zivkovic, Angela M. et al. "Dietary Omega-3 Fatty Acids Aid in the Modulation of Inflammation and Metabolic Health." *California Agriculture* 65.3 (2011): 106–11. https://www.ncbi.nlm.nih.gov/pmc/articles/ PMC4030645/.

13. Campos, Marcelo. "Leaky gut: What is it, and what does it mean for you?" *Harvard Health Blog*, September 22, 2017. https://www.health.harvard.edu/ blog/leaky-gut-what-is-it-and-what-does-it-mean-for-you-2017092212451.

14. Ibid.

15. Thomas Jefferson University. "Stronger intestinal barrier may prevent cancer in the rest of the body, new study suggests." *ScienceDaily*, February 21, 2012. https://www.sciencedaily.com/releases/2012/02/120221212345.htm.

16. Katz, David. "Fortification Follies: Lipstick on a Pig for Breakfast, Lunch and Dinner." *Huffington Post,* April 9, 2014. https://www.huffingtonpost.com/ david-katz-md/diet-and-nutrition_b_4744951.html.

Chapter 10

1. Taleb, N. N. et al (2014). "The precautionary principle (with application to the genetic modification of organisms)." arXiv:1410.5787. https://arxiv.org/ abs/1410.5787.

2. Alsadek, Jihad. "Updated Screening Level Usage Analysis (SLUA) Report for Glyphosate Case PC #s (103601, 103604, 103607, 103608, 103613, and 417300)." Memorandum. Washington, DC: U.S. Environmental Protection Agency, 2015. https://d3n8a8pro7vhmx.cloudfront.net/yesmaam/ pages/680/attachments/original/1492450468/GLYPHOSATE_use_10-22-15. pdf?1492450468.

3. UC San Diego Health. "Exposure to Glyphosate, Chemical Found in Weed Killers, Increased Over 23 Years." News release, October 24, 2017. https:// health.ucsd.edu/news/releases/Pages/2017-10-24-exposure-to-glyphosate -chemical-found-in-weed-killer-increased-over-23-years.aspx.

4. Johnson, Nathanael. "Roundup-ready, aim, spray: How GM crops lead to herbicide addiction." *Grist,* October 14, 2013, Food section. https://grist.org/ food/roundup-ready-aim-spray-how-gm-crops-lead-to-herbicide-addiction/.

5. Pandey, Aparamita and Medhamurthy Rudraiah. "Analysis of Endocrine Disruption Effect of Roundup® in Adrenal Gland of Male Rats." *Toxicology Reports* 2 (2015): 1075–85. https://www.sciencedirect.com/science/article/ pii/S221475001530041X.

6. Thongprakaisang, Siriporn et al. "Glyphosate induces human breast cancer cells growth via estrogen receptors." *Food and Chemical Toxicology* 59 (2013): 129–36. https://www.researchgate.net/publication/237146763_Glyphosate_induces_human_breast_cancer_cells_growth_via_estrogen_receptors.

7. Neslen, "Glyphosate shown to disrupt microbiome 'at safe levels', study claims." *The Guardian.*

8. Schubert, David. "The Coming Food Disaster." CNN, January 28, 2015, Opinion section. https://www.cnn.com/2015/01/27/opinion/schubert-herbicides-crops/index.html.

9. In Re: Roundup Products Liability Litigation,16-md-02741-VC (N.D. Cal. 2016); Baum, Hedlund, Aristei Goldman. "Monsanto Papers | Secret Documents." https://www.baumhedlundlaw.com/toxic-tort-law/monsanto-roundup-lawsuit/monsanto-secret-documents/;_Baum, Hedlund, Aristei Goldman. "monsanto-documents-chart-101217." http://baumhedlundlaw.com/pdf/monsanto-documents/monsanto-documents-chart-101217.pdf.

10. Ibid.

11. Ibid.

12. Gillam, Carey. "Internal EPA Documents Show Scramble For Data On Monsanto's Roundup Herbicide." *Huffington Post*, August 7, 2017. https://www.huffingtonpost.com/entry/internal-epa-documents-show-scramble-for-data-on-monsantos_us_5988dd73e4b030f0e267c6cd.

13. International Agency for Research on Cancer, "Agents Classified by the IARC Monographs, Volumes 1–121."

14. Gillam, Carey. "IARC Scientists Defend Glyphosate Cancer Link; Surprised by Industry Assault." *Huffington Post,* December 6, 2017. https://www.huffingtonpost.com/carey-gillam/iarc-scientists-defend-gl_b_12720306.html.

15. International Agency for Research on Cancer. "IARC response to criticisms of the Monographs and the glyphosate evaluation." http://www.iarc.fr/en/media-centre/iarcnews/pdf/IARC_response_to_criticisms_of_the_Monographs_and_the_glyphosate_evaluation.pdf.

16. Gillam, "IARC Scientists Defend Glyphosate Cancer Link," December 6, 2017.

17. Sesana, Laura. "EPA Raises Levels Of Glyphosate Residue Allowed In Food." *The Washington Times*, July 5, 2013. Archived version: https://web.archive.org/web/20140428230405/http://communities.washingtontimes.com/neighborhood/world-our-backyard/2013/jul/5/epa-raises-levels-glyphosate-residue-allowed-your-/.

18. In Re: Roundup Products Liability Litigation.

19. Rosenblatt, Joel et al. "EPA Official Accused of Helping Monsanto 'Kill' Cancer Study." *Bloomberg*, March 14, 2017. https://www.bloomberg.com/news/articles/2017-03-14/monsanto-accused-of-ghost-writing-papers-on-roundup-cancer-risk.

20. Gillam, Carey. "Questions about EPA-Monsanto collusion raised in cancer lawsuits." *Huffington Post*, February 14, 2018. https://www.huffingtonpost.com/carey-gillam/questions-about-epa-monsa_b_14727648.html.

21. Polansek, Tom. "U.S. EPA says glyphosate not likely to be carcinogenic to people." *Reuters*.

22. Murphy, D. and H. Rowlands. "Glyphosate: Unsafe on Any Plate." Food Democracy Now! and The Detox Project. https://s3.amazonaws.com/media.fooddemocracynow.org/images/FDN_Glyphosate_FoodTesting_Report_p2016.pdf.

23. Gillam, Carey. "Canadians Report Weed Killer Detected in 30 Percent of Food Tested." U.S. Right to Know, April 12, 2017. https://usrtk.org/our-investigations/seek-and-ye-shall-find-canadians-report-weed-killer-detected-in-30-percent-of-food-tested/?mc_cid=2584e742b5&mc_eid=47556c3c3b.

24. Gillam, Carey. "Regulators may recommend testing food for glyphosate residues." *Reuters*, April 20, 2015. https://www.reuters.com/article/us-food-agriculture-glyphosate-idUSKBN0NB1N020150420.

25. Gillam, Carey. "FDA Finds Monsanto's Weed Killer In U.S. Honey." *Huffington Post*, September 16, 2017. https://www.huffingtonpost.com/carey-gillam/fda-finds-monsantos-weed_b_12008680.html.

Chapter 11

1. Rodale Institute. "About Us." https://rodaleinstitute.org/about-us/mission-and-history/.

2. Ibid.

3. Shanker, Deena. "Buying organic veggies at the supermarket is a waste of money." *Quartz*, August 29, 2015. https://qz.com/488851/buying-organic-veggies-at-the-supermarket-is-basically-a-waste-of-money/.

4. Miller, Henry. "The USDA 'Organic' Label Misleads and Rips Off Consumers." *Forbes*, March 7, 2016, Opinion section. https://geneticliteracyproject.org/2016/03/07/the-usda-organic-label-misleads-and-rips-off-consumers/.

5. Krasny, Jill. "Economist Tyler Cowen Says Organic Foods Are Just A 'Marketing Label.'" *Business Insider,* September 19, 2012. http://www.businessinsider.com/economist-organic-foods-just-marketing-2012-9.

6. Burke, Cindy. "Don't Believe the (Organic) Hype." *Tell Me More*. Podcast, June 21, 2007; https://www.npr.org/templates/story/story.php?storyId=11251576.

7. Pamplin Media Group. "Smart Money: Is organic food worth the higher price? Experts say no." *Portland Tribune (Newberg Graphic)*, February 15, 2017, News section. https://portlandtribune.com/nbg/142-news/345111-225219-smart-money-is-organic-food-worth-the-higher-price-experts-say-no.

8. Hamerschlag, Lappé, and Malkan, "Spinning Food."

9. Ibid.

10. Ibid.

11. Hatfield, Jenna. "From Panels to Parties to Sponsors, BlogHer Food '13 Attendees Share It All." *BlogHer*, June 24, 2013. http://www.blogher.com/panels-parties-sponsors-blogher-food-13-attendees-share-it-all.

12. Lappé, Anna. "Big Food uses mommy bloggers to shape public opinion." *Al Jazeera America*, August 1, 2014, Opinion section. http://america.aljazeera.com/opinions/2014/8/food-agriculturemonsantogmoadvertising.html.

13. Aubrey, Allison. "Are Organic Tomatoes Better?" *NPR*, May 29, 2008, Your Health section. https://www.npr.org/templates/story/story.php?storyId=90914182.

14. Oliveira, Aurelice B. et al. "The Impact of Organic Farming on Quality of Tomatoes Is Associated to Increased Oxidative Stress during Fruit Development." *PLOS ONE* 8, no. 2 (February 20, 2013): e56354. https://www.ncbi.nlm.nih.gov/pubmed/23437115.

15. Barański, M. et al. "Higher Antioxidant and Lower Cadmium Concentrations and Lower Incidence of Pesticide Residues in Organically Grown Crops: a Systematic Literature Review and Meta-Analyses." *British Journal of Nutrition* 112, no. 5 (2014): 794–811. https://www.ncbi.nlm.nih.gov/pubmed/24968103.

16. Średnicka-Tober, Dominika et al. "Higher PUFA and n-3 PUFA, Conjugated Linoleic Acid, α-Tocopherol and Iron, but Lower Iodine and Selenium Concentrations in Organic Milk: a Systematic Literature Review and Meta- and Redundancy Analyses." *British Journal of Nutrition* 115, no. 6 (2016): 1043–60. https://www.ncbi.nlm.nih.gov/pubmed/26878105.

17. Holtcamp, Wendee. "Obesogens: An Environmental Link to Obesity." *Environmental Health Perspectives* 120.2 (2012): a62–a68. https://www.ncbi.nlm.nih.gov/pmc/articles/PMC3279464/.

18. Baillie-Hamilton, Paula. "Chemical Toxins: A Hypothesis to Explain the Global Obesity Epidemic." *The Journal of Alternative and Complementary Medicine* 8, no. 2 (April 2002): 185–92. https://www.ncbi.nlm.nih.gov/pubmed/12006126.

19. Kristof, "Warnings from a Flabby Mouse," *New York Times*.

20. Harvard T. H. Chan School of Public Health. "Health benefits of organic food, farming outlined in new report." https://www.hsph.harvard.edu/news/features/health-benefits-organic-food-farming-report/.

21. Barański et al, "Higher Antioxidant and Lower Cadmium Concentrations and Lower Incidence of Pesticide Residues in Organically Grown Crops," 794–811.

22. Pesticide Action Network North America, What's On My Food. "How Much Is Too Much?" http://www.whatsonmyfood.org/howmuch.jsp.

23. Roberts, J. R. and C. J. Karr, Council on Environmental Health. "Pesticide Exposure in Children." *Pediatrics* 130, issue 6 (2012): e1765–88. https://www.ncbi.nlm.nih.gov/pubmed/23184105.

24. Greene, Ronnie. "Poisoning Workers at the Bottom of the Food Chain." *Mother Jones*, June 25, 2012, Environment section. https://www.motherjones.com/environment/2012/06/pesticides-farm-workers-poison-epa/.

25. Reuben, S. "2008–2009 Annual Report President's Cancer Panel. Reducing Environmental Cancer Risk: What We Can Do Now." National Cancer Institute. https://deainfo.nci.nih.gov/advisory/pcp/annualreports/pcp08 -09rpt/pcp_report_08-09_508.pdf.

26. Ibid.

27. National Institute of Environmental Health Sciences, "Endocrine Disruptors," May 2010.

28. United Nations Human Rights. "Pesticides are 'global human rights concern,' say UN experts urging new treaty." News release, March 7, 2017. Office of the United Nations High Commissioner for Human Rights. http:// www.ohchr.org/EN/NewsEvents/Pages/DisplayNews.aspx?NewsID=21306.

29. Ibid.

30. U.S. Department of Agriculture. "Organic Labeling Standards." https:// www.ams.usda.gov/grades-standards/organic-labeling-standards.

31. U.S. Department of Agriculture. "Organic Regulations." https://www.ams .usda.gov/rules-regulations/organic.

32 Pesticide Action Network North America. What's On My Food? "Pesticides: A Public Problem." http://www.whatsonmyfood.org/index.jsp.

33. Eng, Monica. "Another concern: Drug residues in meat." *Chicago Tribune*, May 26, 2013, News section. http:// articles.chicagotribune.com/2013-05-26/news/ ct-met-antibiotics-residue-20130526_1_u-s-meat-the-fda-drug-violations.

34. Environmental Working Group. "EWG's 2018 Shopper's Guide to Pesticides in Produce," Dirty Dozen. https://www.ewg.org/foodnews/dirty-dozen .php; Environmental Working Group. "OUT NOW: EWG's 2018 Shopper's Guide to Pesticides in Produce." https://www.ewg.org/foodnews/press.php.

Chapter 12

1. Fiolet, Thibault, et al. "Consumption of ultra-processed foods and cancer risk: results from NutriNet-Santé prospective cohort." *BMJ* 360 (February 2018): k322. https://doi.org/10.1136/bmj.k322.

Bonus Section

1. National Cancer Institute. "Cruciferous Vegetables and Cancer Prevention." https://www.cancer.gov/about-cancer/causes-prevention/risk/diet/ cruciferous-vegetables-fact-sheet.

2. Wallig, M. et al. "Synergy among Phytochemicals within Crucifers: Does It Translate into Chemoprotection?" *The Journal of Nutrition* 135, issue 12 (2005): 2972S–2977S. https://academic.oup.com/jn/ article/135/12/2972S/4669948.

3. Christensen, K. L. Y. et al. "The contribution of diet to total bisphenol A body burden in humans: Results of a 48 hour fasting study." *Environment International* 50 (2012): 7–14. https://www.ncbi.nlm.nih.gov/pubmed/23026348.

4. Wilson, Clare. "Calorie restriction diet extends life of monkeys by years." *New Scientist*, January 2017. https://www.newscientist.com/article/2118224-calorie-restriction-diet-extends-life-of-monkeys-by-years/; Healy, Melissa. "Longer fasts might help with weight loss but Americans eat all day long." *Los Angeles Times*, September 24, 2015. http://www.latimes.com/science/sciencenow/la-sci-sn-americans-all-day-eating-20150924-story.html.

5. MacIntosh, A. "The effects of a short program of detoxification in disease-free individuals." *Alternative Therapies in Health and Medicine*, July 1, 2000, 6(4):70–76. https://europepmc.org/abstract/med/10895516.

6. Rodriguez, T. Saénz et al. "Choleretic activity and biliary elimination of lipids and bile acids induced by an artichoke leaf extract in rats." *Phytomedicine* 9, no. 8 (2002): 687–93. https://doi.org/10.1078/094471102321621278.

7. Krajka-Kuźniak, Violetta et al. "Betanin, a Beetroot Component, Induces Nuclear Factor Erythroid-2-Related Factor 2-Mediated Expression of Detoxifying/Antioxidant Enzymes in Human Liver Cell Lines." *British Journal of Nutrition* 110, no. 12 (2013): 2138–49. https://www.ncbi.nlm.nih.gov/pubmed/23769299.

8. Munday, R. et al. "Comparative effects of mono-, di-, tri-, and tetrasulfides derived from plants of the Allium family: redox cycling in vitro and hemolytic activity and Phase 2 enzyme induction in vivo." *Free Radic Biol Med.* 34, issue 9 (2003): 1200–1211. http://europepmc.org/abstract/MED/12706500.

9. Wang, E., and M. Wink. "Chlorophyll enhances oxidative stress tolerance in Caenorhabditis elegans and extends its lifespan." *PeerJ* 4 (2016): e1879. https://peerj.com/articles/1879/.

10. Park, Kun-Young et al. "Health Benefits of Kimchi (Korean Fermented Vegetables) as a Probiotic Food." *Journal of Medicinal Food* 17, issue 1 (2014). https://www.ncbi.nlm.nih.gov/pubmed/24456350.

11. Wallig, M. "Synergy among Phytochemicals within Crucifers: Does It Translate into Chemoprotection?" *The Journal of Nutrition* 135, issue 12 (2005): 2972S–2977S.

12. Perez, Jose L. et al. "In Vivo induction of Phase II Detoxifying Enzymes, Glutathione Transferase and Quinone Reductase by Citrus Triterpenoids." *BMC Complementary and Alternative Medicine* 10 (2010): 51. https://www.ncbi.nlm.nih.gov/pmc/articles/PMC2954937/.

13. Healthline. "Top 11 Science-Based Health Benefits of Pumpkin Seeds." https://www.healthline.com/nutrition/11-benefits-of-pumpkin-seeds.

Appendix

1. Center for Science in the Public Interest. "Chemical Cuisine: Acesulfame Potassium." https://cspinet.org/eating-healthy/chemical-cuisine#acesulfamek.

2. Yang, Qing. "Gain Weight by 'Going Diet?' Artificial Sweeteners and the Neurobiology of Sugar Cravings: Neuroscience 2010." *The Yale Journal of Biology and Medicine* 83.2 (2010): 101–8. https://www.ncbi.nlm.nih.gov/pmc/articles/PMC2892765/.

3. Soffritti, Morando et al. "First Experimental Demonstration of the Multipotential Carcinogenic Effects of Aspartame Administered in the Feed to Sprague-Dawley Rats." *Environmental Health Perspectives* 114.3 (2006): 379–85. https://www.ncbi.nlm.nih.gov/pmc/articles/PMC1392232/; Ferrari, Nancy. "Is there a link between diet soda and heart disease?" *Harvard Health Blog*, February 21, 2012. https://www.health.harvard.edu/blog/is-there-a-link-between-diet-soda-and-heart-disease-201202214296.

4. Jing Ye et al. "Assessment of the Determination of Azodicarbonamide and Its Decomposition Product Semicarbazide: Investigation of Variation in Flour and Flour Products." *Journal of Agricultural and Food Chemistry* 59, no. 17 (2011): 9313–18. https://www.ncbi.nlm.nih.gov/pubmed/21786817.

5. Lefferts, Lisa. "FDA Should Ban Azodicarbonamide, Says CSPI." Center for Science in the Public Interest, February 4, 2014. https://cspinet.org/new/201402041.html.

6. Ibid.

7. Environmental Working Group. "EWG's Dirty Dozen Guide to Food Additives." https://www.ewg.org/research/ewg-s-dirty-dozen-guide-food-additives/generally-recognized-as-safe-but-is-it#.W4hygpNKiRs.

8. Lefferts, "FDA Should Ban Azodicarbonamide, Says CSPI."

9. Environmental Working Group, "EWG's Dirty Dozen Guide to Food Additives."

10. Henriques, Martha. "Additive in breakfast cereals could make the brain 'forget' to stop eating." *International Business Times*, August 10, 2017. http://www.ibtimes.co.uk/additive-breakfast-cereals-could-make-brain-forget-stop-eating-1634413.

11. Bryce, Martha. "Hues of Blues in the News: Blue dye in foods present health concerns." *WhyDye?* (Blog), January 17, 2013. http://www.whydye.org/2013/01/hues-of-blues-in-the-news-health-concerns-of-ingesting-artificial-blue-dye/.

12. Kobylewski and Jacobson, "Food Dyes: A Rainbow of Risks."

13. Dengate, S. and A. Ruben. "Controlled trial of cumulative behavioural effects of a common bread preservative." *Journal of Paediatrics and Child Health* 38 (2002): 373–76. https://www.ncbi.nlm.nih.gov/pubmed/12173999.

14. Charlton, K. M. et al. "Cardiac Lesions in Rats Fed Rapeseed Oils." *Canadian Journal of Comparative Medicine* 39, no. 3 (1975): 261–69. https://www.ncbi .nlm.nih.gov/pmc/articles/PMC1277456/.

15. O'Keefe, S., et al. "Levels Of Transgeometrical Isomers Of Essential Fatty Acids In Some Unhydrogenated U. S. Vegetable Oils." *Journal of Food Lipids* 1 (1994): 165–76. https://onlinelibrary.wiley.com/doi/ abs/10.1111/j.1745-4522.1994.tb00244.x; Fallon, Sally and Mary G. Enig. "The Great Con-ola." The Weston A. Price Foundation, July 28, 2002. https://www.westonaprice.org/health-topics/know-your-fats/ the-great-con-ola/.

16. International Agency for Research on Cancer, "Agents Classified by the IARC Monographs, Volumes 1–121."

17. Walsh, Bryan. "Do the Chemicals That Turn Soda Brown Also Cause Cancer?" *Time*, February 17, 2011. http://healthland.time.com/2011/02/17/ do-the-chemicals-that-turn-soda-brown-also-cause-cancer/; Center for Science in the Public Interest. "Petition to bar the use of caramel colorings produced with ammonia and containing certain carcinogens." February 16, 2011. https://cspinet.org/resource/petition-bar-use-caramel-colorings -produced-ammonia-and-containing-certain-carcinogens.

18. Ciriminna, Rosaria et al. "Citric Acid: Emerging Applications of Key Biotechnology Industrial Product." *Chemistry Central Journal* 11 (2017): 22. https://ccj.springeropen.com/articles/10.1186/s13065-017-0251-y.

19. Rodale Institute. "Chemical cotton." February 4, 2014. http://rodaleinstitute .org/chemical-cotton/.

20. Environmental Justice Foundation in collaboration with Pesticide Action. "The Deadly Chemicals in Cotton." 2007. https://ejfoundation.org// resources/downloads/the_deadly_chemicals_in_cotton.pdf.

21. Hardin, Pete. "FDA Approved Polydimethylsiloxane in Foods in 1998." *The Milkweed*, March 2006. http://www.themilkweed.com/Pizza_Cheese _Update_March_2006.pdf.

22. Van den Broeck, Hetty C. et al. "Presence of Celiac Disease Epitopes in Modern and Old Hexaploid Wheat Varieties: Wheat Breeding May Have Contributed to Increased Prevalence of Celiac Disease." *Theoretical and Applied Genetics.* 121.8 (2010): 1527–39. https://www.ncbi.nlm.nih.gov/ pubmed/20664999.

23. Price, Annie. "Erythritol: The Good, the Bad & the Ugly with This Common Sweetener." Dr. Axe, October 12, 2016. https://draxe.com/erythritol/.

24. Kresser, Chris. "Harmful or Harmless: Guar Gum, Locust Bean Gum, and More." *Chris Kresser (Blog)*, December 13, 2013. https://chriskresser.com/ harmful-or-harmless-guar-gum-locust-bean-gum-and-more/.

25. Hyman, Mark. "5 Reasons High Fructose Corn Syrup Will Kill You." *Mark Hyman, M.D.* (Blog), https://drhyman.com/ blog/2011/05/13/5-reasons-high-fructose-corn-syrup-will-kill-you/.

26. American Chemical Society. "Soda Warning? High-Fructose Corn Syrup Linked To Diabetes, New Study Suggests." *ScienceDaily*, August 23, 2007. https://www.sciencedaily.com/releases/2007/08/070823094819.htm.

27. Dufault, Renee et al. "Mercury from chlor-alkali plants: measured concentrations in product sugar." *Environmental Health*. 8 (2009):2. https://ehjournal.biomedcentral.com/articles/10.1186/1476-069X-8-2.

28. Cleveland Clinic. "Researcher Links Digestive Problems to Food Additive." https://giving.clevelandclinic.org/articles/researcher-links-digestive-problems-food-additive.

29. Nutrition for Optimal Health Association. "Review of: Excitotoxins: The Taste that Kills." *Nutrition Digest* 38, No. 2 (1995). http://americannutritionassociation.org/newsletter/review-excitotoxins-taste-kills.

30. Environmental Working Group, "Synthetic Ingredients in Natural Flavors and Natural Flavors in Artificial Flavors."

31. Mercola, Joseph. "Neotame: Is This More-Dangerous-than-Aspartame Sweetener Hiding in Your Food?" March 28, 2012. http://articles.mercola.com/sites/articles/archive/2012/03/28/neotame-more-toxic-than-aspartame.aspx.

32. Charles, A. K. and P. D. Darbre. "Combinations of parabens at concentrations measured in human breast tissue can increase proliferation of MCF-7 human breast cancer cells." *Journal of Applied Toxicology* 33 (2013): 390–98. https://onlinelibrary.wiley.com/doi/abs/10.1002/jat.2850;_Khanna S., P. R. Dash, and P. D. Darbre. "Exposure to parabens at the concentration of maximal proliferative response increases migratory and invasive activity of human breast cancer cells in vitro." *J. Appl. Toxicol.* 34 (2014): 1051–59. https://onlinelibrary.wiley.com/doi/abs/10.1002/jat.3003.

33. Willett, Walter and Dariush Mozaffarian. "Trans fats in cardiac and diabetes risk: An overview." *Current Cardiovascular Risk Reports* 1 (2007): 16–23. https://link.springer.com/article/10.1007%2Fs12170-007-0004-x.

34. Environmental Working Group, "EWG's Dirty Dozen Guide to Food Additives."

35. Kobylewski and Jacobson, "Food Dyes: A Rainbow of Risks."

36. Ibid.

37. Bøhn, Thomas et al. "Compositional differences in soybeans on the market: Glyphosate accumulates in Roundup Ready GM soybeans." *Food Chemistry* 153 (2014): 207–15. https://www.sciencedirect.com/science/article/pii/S0308814613019201.

38. Gupta, Raj Kishor, Shivraj Singh Gangoliya, and Nand Kumar Singh. "Reduction of Phytic Acid and Enhancement of Bioavailable Micronutrients in Food Grains." *Journal of Food Science and Technology* 52.2 (2015): 676–84. https://www.ncbi.nlm.nih.gov/pmc/articles/PMC4325021/.

39. Coca-Cola Company. "Rebaudioside A Composition and Method for Purifying Rebaudioside A." United States Patent Application 20070292582, December 20, 2007. http://appft.uspto.gov/netacgi/nph-Parser?Sect1=PTO2&Sect2=HITOFF&p=1&u=%2Fnetahtml%2FPTO%2Fsearch-bool.html&r=2&f=G&l=50&col=AND&d=PG01&s1=11751627&OS=11751627&RS=11751627.

40. Center for Science in the Public Interest, "CSPI Downgrades Sucralose from 'Caution' to 'Avoid,'" February. 8, 2016.

41. Kelley, Geri and Sarina Gleason. "Common Additive May Be Why You Have Food Allergies." *Michigan State University*, July 11, 2016. http://msutoday.msu.edu/news/2016/common-additive-may-be-why-you-have-food-allergies/.

42. Illuminato, Ian. "Tiny Ingredients, Big Risks." *Friends of the Earth U.S.*, May 2014. https://1bps6437gg8c169i0y1drtgz-wpengine.netdna-ssl.com/wp-content/uploads/wpallimport/files/archive/2014_Tiny_Ingredients_Big_Risks_Web.pdf.

43. Kobylewski and Jacobson, "Food Dyes: A Rainbow of Risks."

44. Ibid.

Index

A

Abbott (drug company), 29
academia, 11–17, 88–89, 92–96, 114
Academy of Nutrition and Dietetics, 17
acesulfame potassium (Ace-K, Equal), 109, 125, 231
activism and activists
  against food additives, xi, xix–xx, 61–62, 105–108
  discrediting, by Big Food industry, xi–xiii, 42–44, 115–116
  mission of, xv–xix, xxi
added sugars
  to cereals, 153–154, 166
  to "fat-free" products, 30, 84, 124, 126–127
  in gluten-free products, 133
  to herbal-fortified beverages, 162
  probiotics and, 165
  types of, 101
addictions and cravings
  to artificial sweeteners, 66, 103
  Big Food industry on, 146–147
  food tracking for fighting, 116–117
  to natural flavors, 141–142, 144–147
  to soda, 111–112, 116–118
  to sugar, 84–85, 91, 98–99, 101, 102–103
  to "sugar-free" foods, 125–126
advanced glycation end products (AGEs), 86
Ag Canada, 29
Agri-Pulse, on GMO animal feed use, 9–10
Ajinomoto, 71
Allen, Will, 12
Alliance for Food and Farming, 38, 180
"all natural" labeling, 122, 123

Amarin, 28–29
American Academy of Pediatrics, 113, 189–190
American Association of University Professors, 15
American Beverage Association, 10, 111, 112–113
American Council on Science and Health (ACSH), 7–8
American Diabetes Association, 83, 113
American Egg Board (AEB), 19–20
American Farm Bureau Federation, 9
American food ingredients. *See also* ingredient evaluation, of packaged foods
  action steps for, 61–62
  European vs., 53–57
  processed food testing and, 58–61. *See also* U.S. Food and Drug Administration
  U.S. health statistics and, 57–58
American Heart Association (AHA), 27–31, 83, 113
American Journal of Clinical Nutrition (AJCN), on processed foods, 16
American Journal of Preventive Medicine, on soda industry's funding, 113
American Seed Trade Association, 13, 35
American Society of Nutrition (ASN), 16
Amgen, 28–29
ancient grains, 134
Anheuser-Bush petition, 26
animal feed, 9–10, 96, 194
animal proteins. *See* meats
Annals of Internal Medicine, on sugar consumption, 88–89
Annie's Chocolate Bunnies, 144–145
Annual Reviews of Public Health, diet recommendations by, 78

Godoy, Maria, 32–36
goiters (thyroid), 155–156
The Good Food Revolution (Allen), 12
"a good source of fiber" labeling, 122, 124
"grain-free" labeling, 136
grains
    about: detoxifying choices, 215–216, 220, 229; fortification of, 156; gluten-free options, 134–135; labeling, 29, 122, 123–124, 134, 136; as nutrients source, 166; whole grains, 133, 134–135, 166
    Quinoa Stir-fry, 224
Grandjean, Philippe, 188
GRAS ("Generally Recognized as Safe"), 59–61, 143–144
Great Lakes Crop Summit, 35
Grocery Manufacturers Association, 9, 10
guar gum, 239
gut bacteria (microbiome), 69–70, 77–78, 102, 132, 164, 171

H

Hampton Creek (vegan food startup), 20
Harvard University, 30, 81–82, 92
Hawaii, 42–43
Hawaii Center for Food Safety (Hawaii CFS), 42–43
"health" foods. *See also* low-calorie processed foods
    flavored waters as soda alternatives, 109–110
    sugars in, 83, 89–90, 126–127, 129, 132, 133
health policy. *See* U.S. Centers for Disease Control and Prevention; U.S. Department of Agriculture; U.S. Food and Drug Administration
healthy fats, 100, 127
heart health, 87, 108–109, 126
Heinz Tomato Ketchup, 56
hemp seeds, 100. *See also* nuts and seeds
Henderson, Elizabeth, 8
herb-drug interactions, 163–164
Hershey's, 9, 17, 88
hexane, 185
HFCS-90 (fructose or fructose syrup), 97, 239–240

high-fructose corn syrup (HFCS), 75, 97, 239
Hint flavored water, 142–143
hippocampus, 86–87
honey, 103.
    See also natural sweeteners
Horizon Organic Lowfat Chocolate Milk, 161
hormone-treated dairy, 75
Humira, 45
Hyman, Mark, 65, 85

I

I Can't Believe It's Not Butter, light version, 128
ice cream, 94–95
imitation vanilla, 247
Infante, Peter, 22
inflammation, 86, 164–165
ingredient evaluation, of packaged foods, 197–205, 231–248. *See also specific ingredients*
    about, 197–198
    to avoid at all costs, 231–248
    calorie quality and, 200–201
    ingredient lists, 198–199
    source of, 201–205
Institute of Food Technologists, 35
Institute of Medicine and the National Research Council, 57
insulin and insulin resistance, 65, 67, 76, 87–88, 125
International Agency for Research on Cancer (IARC), 107, 132, 172–173, 235
International Life Sciences Institute (ILSI), 88–89, 111, 115
International Service for the Acquisition of Agri-biotech Applications, 8
iodized salt, 156
"Is the Food Babe a Fearmonger? Scientists Are Speaking Out" (Godoy), 32–35

J

Jenny Craig diet, 73–74
Jif peanut butter, 127
journalists, 6–7, 8–9

leaky gut syndrome and, 164–165
weight loss and, 95–96
propaganda, 3–23. *See also* biased
media; "health" foods
about, 3–5, 23
academia and, 11–14
by academics, 11–14
of front groups, 5–7
front groups and, 5–7
lobbying as, 18–22
for low-calorie processed foods, 71–72
New York Times exposé on, 14
nutrition experts and, 17–18, 25–26
sponsored research as, 14–17
on sugar consumption, 88–89
of trade groups, 10
trade groups and associations as,
10–11
propyl gallate, 242
propylparaben (E216), 242
protein bars, 89
Pumpkin Spice Latte (Starbucks), xi,
xiii, 105–108
Pure, White, and Deadly (Yudkin),
82–83
Purely Elizabeth Ancient Grain Granola, 167

Q

Qi'a Superfood cereals, 167
QR codes, 20–21
Quaker Oats products, 56
Quinoa Stir-fry, 224

R

ractopamine, 186
real foods. *See* whole foods
"real fruit" labeling, 90, 122, 124
Red #3 (erythrosine), 243
Red #40 (allura red), 53, 56–57, 110, 243
"reduced fat" labeling, 127
refined oils, 127–128
refined sugars
alternatives to, 200–201
in breakfast cereals, 95–96
gut health and, 164–165
in "health" foods, 89–90, 126–127,
129, 132, 133

inflammation and, 86, 164–165
types of, 4, 69, 237
weight gain and, 94
Regeneron/Sanofi, 29
research, sponsored, 14–17, 88–89,
92–96, 114, 143–144
restaurants, dining out at, 203–204. *See
also specific restaurants*
Rice Krispies, 62, 167
rice starch, 132
Rodale, J. I., 177–178
Rosenbloom, Cara, 37–38
rotenone, 192
Roundup weed killer, 169–176
about, 169–171
action steps against, 175–176
defense of, 34, 172–174
organic crop ban on, 183
Rowland, Jess, 174
Rudkin, Margaret, xvi–xviii
RXBARS, 129, 139–140

S

sabotage, 42–44
saccharin, 66
saccharin (Sweet'N Low), 66, 103, 125
salad dressings
about, 90
Coconut Oil Dressing, 224
salads
for gluten-free diet, 135
Simple Avocado Salad, 225
The Salt (blog), 32–36
Sargento shredded cheese, 129
sauerkraut, 102. *See also* fermented foods
Schatzker, Mark, 144–145, 150–151, 152
Schlatter, James, 66
Schubert, Dave, 171
Schwarcz, Joe, xiv
seeds. *See* nuts and seeds
Senapathy, Kavin, 33–34
Sensient Technologies Corporation, xiii
serotonin, 102
sewage sludge, 185–186, 192
Simon, Michele, 15–16
60 Minutes interview, on food addiction, 146–147
Skinny Cow ice cream sandwiches,
68–69
skipping meals, 100
sleep habits, 102

Y

Yellow #5 (tartrazine), 53, 56, 110, 248
Yellow #6 (sunset yellow), 56, 248
yellow dye petitions, 62
yoga mat chemical, 26, 62, 232
yogurt, 67–68, 102, 140. *See also* fermented foods
Yudkin, John, 82–83

Z

"zero" calorie health claims, 109–110
zinc, 159

Acknowledgments

I am forever grateful for my daughter, Harley. She has given me the strength, the fortitude, and the motivation to share the lessons in this book with the world. My greatest hope is that her generation becomes wise to the ways of the food industry and they achieve the best health imaginable.

To my husband, Finley, who makes all my dreams come true and a book possible with his incredible encouragement and support.

As I continue my career as a food activist, and now a food company owner, my family has been there every step of the way. To my grandparents, Mom, Dad, Father-in-law Finley, Mother-in-law Diane, Laura, Yog, Judy, Ian and Dylan, Summers, Henry, and Taylor, thank you for the love and laughter.

To Sushila Melvani and the Sri Aurobindo Society in Pondicherry, India, for looking after me, praying for me, and sending blessings throughout my life.

Thank you to Kim and Pam for being the most loyal, dedicated, and hardworking team. To Derek, Devin, Melanie, and everyone at Truvani for supporting my mission and the book launch.

To my two brilliant agents, Steve Troha and Scott Hoffman. I'll never forget the moment the title for this book was born and the conversations we had about it. To the entire Hay House team for guiding me and making this book possible. To my editors Mary Norris, Sally Mason-Swaab, Anne Barthel, and Maggie Greenwood Robinson, for helping me to make this book rock solid.

Last but not least, to all the food activists who have come before me, including Gary Ruskin, Stacy Malkan, Carey Gillam, Max Goldberg, John Roulac, and Zuri Allen.

To all my inspiring readers. Thanks for sticking by my side and spreading the truth despite all the mudslinging. "No Mud No Lotus."

About the Author

Named as one of the most influential people on the Internet by *Time* magazine, Vani Hari is a food activist, *New York Times* best-selling author of *The Food Babe Way*, and co-founder of Truvani. For most of her life, Vani ate whatever she wanted—candy, soda, fast food, processed food—until her typical American diet landed her where that diet typically does, in a hospital. Despite her successful career in corporate consulting, Hari decided that health had to become a priority. Her newfound goal drove her to investigate what is really in our food, how it is grown, and what chemicals are used in its production. The more she learned, the more she changed and the better she felt.

Encouraged by her friends and family, Hari started a blog called foodbabe.com in 2011. It quickly became a massive vehicle for change. Foodbabe.com has led campaigns against food giants like Kraft, Starbucks, Chick-fil-A, Subway, and General Mills that attracted more than 500,000 signatures and led to the removal of several controversial ingredients used by these companies. Through corporate activism, petitions, and social media campaigns, Hari and her Food Babe Army have become one of the most powerful populist forces in the health and food industries. Her drive to change the food system inspired the creation of her new company, called Truvani, where she produces real food without added chemicals, products without toxins, and labels without lies. Hari has been profiled in *The New York Times* and *USA Today* and has appeared on *Good Morning America*, CNN, *The Dr. Oz Show*, *The Doctors*, and NPR. She lives in Charlotte, North Carolina, with her husband, Finley, and daughter, Harley.

Hay House Titles of Related Interest

YOU CAN HEAL YOUR LIFE, the movie, starring Louise Hay & Friends
(available as a 1-DVD program, an expanded 2-DVD set,
and an online streaming video)
Learn more at www.hayhouse.com/louise-movie

THE SHIFT, the movie, starring Dr. Wayne W. Dyer
(available as a 1-DVD program, an expanded 2-DVD set,
and an online streaming video)
Learn more at www.hayhouse.com/the-shift-movie

■ ■ ■

*THE ALKALINE RESET CLEANSE: The 7-Day Reboot for Unlimited
Energy, Rapid Weight Loss, and the Prevention of Degenerative Disease,*
by Ross Bridgeford

CHRIS BEAT CANCER: A Comprehensive Plan for Healing Naturally,
by Chris Wark

*HEAL YOUR DRAINED BRAIN: Naturally Relieve Anxiety, Combat
Insomnia,* and *Balance Your Brain in Just 14 Days,* by Dr. Mike Dow

*YOUNG AND SLIM FOR LIFE: 10 Essential Steps to Achieve Total Vitality
and Kick-Start Weight Loss That Lasts,* by Frank Lipman, M.D.

All of the above are available at your local bookstore,
or may be ordered by contacting Hay House (see next page).

■ ■ ■

We hope you enjoyed this Hay House book. If you'd like to receive our online catalog featuring additional information on Hay House books and products, or if you'd like to find out more about the Hay Foundation, please contact:

Hay House, Inc., P.O. Box 5100, Carlsbad, CA 92018-5100
(760) 431-7695 or (800) 654-5126
(760) 431-6948 (fax) or (800) 650-5115 (fax)
www.hayhouse.com® • www.hayfoundation.org

———

Published in Australia by:
Hay House Australia Pty. Ltd., 18/36 Ralph St., Alexandria NSW 2015
Phone: 612-9669-4299 • *Fax:* 612-9669-4144 • www.hayhouse.com.au

Published in the United Kingdom by:
Hay House UK, Ltd., Astley House, 33 Notting Hill Gate, London W11 3JQ
Phone: 44-20-3675-2450 • *Fax:* 44-20-3675-2451 • www.hayhouse.co.uk

Published in India by: Hay House Publishers India,
Muskaan Complex, Plot No. 3, B-2, Vasant Kunj, New Delhi 110 070
Phone: 91-11-4176-1620 • *Fax:* 91-11-4176-1630 • www.hayhouse.co.in

———

Access New Knowledge.
Anytime. Anywhere.

Learn and evolve at your own pace
with the world's leading experts.

www.hayhouseU.com

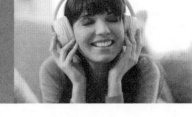